Sailing and Science

– in an Interdisciplinary Perspective

SAILING AND SCIENCE – IN AN INTERDISCIPLINARY PERSPECTIVE
Copyright © Institute of Exercise and Sport Sciences, University of Copenhagen

Editor: Gisela Sjøgaard
Series editor: Jens Bangsbo
Design and layout: Allis Skovbjerg Jepsen
Printed By: Olesen Offset, Viborg
Fotos: *Front:* Charles Sheeler, USA 1948. *Page 18:* Viking Ship Museum, Roskilde. *Page 34, 52, 118:* Gisela Sjøgaard. *Page 76:* Steen Jacobsen, Nordfoto. *Page 94:* Bo Leihof. *Page 130:* Marco Marchetti

ISBN 87 89361 63 6

Institute of Exercise and Sport Sciences
University of Copenhagen
Nørre Allé 51
DK-2200 Copenhagen

Phone: +45 35 32 08 29
Fax: +45 35 32 08 70
e-mail: IFI@ifi.ku.dk
Homepage: www.ifi.ku.dk

This book is supported by The Danish Counsil for Sports Research.

Sailing and Science

– in an Interdisciplinary Perspective

Editor
Gisela Sjøgaard

Series editor
Jens Bangsbo

Institute of Exercise and Sport Sciences
University of Copenhagen

Copenhagen 1999

Content

Preface

In August 1997 the 2nd "European Congress of Sport and Exercise Science" was held in Copenhagen with more than 800 participants. The scientific programme covered all aspects of exercise and sport sciences with more than 100 invited speakers and 400 presentations. Within the theme "Science and Sport" a number of symposia covered sports from a multidiciplinary perspective. As many people have expressed an interest in this multidisciplinary approach of sport we have decided to produce a series of books on soccer, sailing, running and European diversity in sport and physical activity, respectively. We have been fortunate that so many experts have agreed to contribute to the books allowing for an integration of physiological, psychological, historical and social aspects of the sport. Each chapter in the books provides up-to-date knowledge about the topic and includes a high number of references to allow the reader to go further into depth with the subject area. It is anticipated and hoped that the books will be useful for university researchers, teachers and students as well as for interested coaches.

We will like to express our appreciation to the authors and reviewers as well as the editors for their great effort, which has enabled us to produce these informative books.

Jens Bangsbo
Series editor

Preword

The annual congress of the European College of Sports Science was held in Copenhagen, Denmark in 1997. Denmark has a well established reputation in the international arena of ships used for a large variety of activities, ranging from old-time warfare and trade to sports and pleasure. Denmark is among the countries with long coastlines, so nature has so to speak invited the population to conquer the sea. The famous Vikings had a solid platform in Denmark and build sail- and manpowered boats for war and trade. These today have been exchanged with motor driven ships and ferries. Thus the shipyard industry has a long tradition in Denmark, and in spite of major international reconstruction of this industry, the knowledge captured in Denmark is still internationally recognized. Similarly, within sports Danish crews and individual sailors have achieved top positions in competitions. One of the most famous living legends is Paul Elvstrøm, who participated in 8 Olympic Games 1948-1988, the two last teamed up with his daughter Trine, and won Gold Medals in 1948, 1952, 1956 and 1960. Actually, since sailing was included as discipline in the Olympics, Denmark only once did not succeed to win a medal, which was in 1984 in Los Angeles. Most recently Christine Roug impressed at the Olympic Games when she won the Gold medal in 1996. Very good Danish teams are also presently competing internationally e.g. in the discipline of match racing, where two Danish teams are seated within the top 10 of the world match race rankings.

In short, relative to the size of their nation Danes participate in many sailing races and perform remarkable well. Sailing may be considered as one of the national sports, which is also mirrored in the non-elite sailor population, where many enthusiasts spend a major part of their leisure time on the water. Naturally, special interest and knowledge therefore is captured in Denmark.

The above is a background for the organizers to choose this sporting area as one of the central themes of the congress. Further, an original feature of this congress is that it gathers all disciplines relevant to sports science ranging from humanities, social and behavioral sciences over medicine, physiology, and nutrition to biomechanics and technological development. Sailing captures scientific approaches within all these disciplines and thus is the perfect example to demonstrate the interdisciplinary knowledge needed to optimize performance. It was a pleasure to compose a symposium specifically devoted to sailing and to invite for this symposium internationally known capacities in their respective fields. To allow this unique constellation of knowledge to be spread to a larger audience, the lectures have been gathered in this book on „Sailing and Science – in an Interdisciplinary Perspective". I want to thank the authors for their interesting contributions and my colleagues associate professors Ole Lammert and Søren Nagbøll at the Institute of Sports Science and Clinical Biomechanics at the University of Southern Denmark, for assisting me with the review process.

Gisela Sjøgaard
Editor

List of Editors and Authors

JENS BANGSBO, Institute of Exercise and Sport Siences, University of Copenhagen, Universitetsparken 13, DK-2100 Copenhagen Ø, Denmark. Telephone: (+45) 3532 1623 Fax: (+45) 3532 1600 E-mail: JBangsbo@aki.ku.dk

FINN BOJSEN-MØLLER, Laboratory for Functional Anatomy and Biomechanics, University of Copenhagen, Blegdamsvej 3, DK-2200 Copenhagen N, Denmark. Telephone: (+45) 3532 7232 Fax: (+45) 3532 7217 E-mail: F.Moller@mai.ku.dk

OLE CRUMLIN-PEDERSEN, adj. professor, Centre for Maritime Archaeology, Havnevej 7, P.O.Box 317, DK-4000 Roskilde, Denmark. Telephone: (+45) 4632 1600.

ANTONIO DAL MONTE, Prof. M. D., Istituto di Scienza dello Sport, via dei Campi Sportivi 46/48, 00197, Rome, Italy. Telephone: (+39) 6 - 3685 9104 Fax: (+39) 6 - 3685 9221 E-mail: ISS_Fisiologia@coni.it

LEIF HAMBRÆUS, Prof., Dept. of Medical Science, Nutrition unit, Dag Hammarskjölds väg 21, SE-75237 Uppsala, Sweden. Telephone: (+46) 18 471 2211 Fax: (+46) 1855 9505 E-mail: Leif.Hambraeus@nutrition.uu.se

KLAUS HEINEMANN, Professor, Dr., Institute of Sociology, University of Hamburg, Allende-Platz 1, D-20146 Hamburg, Germany. Telephone: (040) 42838-4659/4665 Fax: (040) 42838-3826 E-mail: Heinemann@sozwi.sozialwiss.uni-hamburg.de

MARCO MARCHETTI, Istituto di Fisiologia Umana Facoltà di Medicina e Chirurgia, Università di Roma La Sapienza, Piazza A. Moro 5, 00185 Roma Italy. Telephone: +396 4959256 Fax +396 4452303 E-mail: marchetti@axrma.uniroma1.it

GISELA SJØGAARD, Institute of Sports Science and Clinical Biomechanics, University of Southern Denmark, Campusvej 55, DK-5230 Odense M, Denmark. Telephone: (+45) 6550 3429 Fax: (+45) 6615 8186 E-mail: gis@sportmed.sdu.dk

NEIL SPURWAY, M.A., PhD, Prof., Centre for Exercise Science and Medicine, Institute of Biomedical and Life Sciences, West Medical Building, University of Glasgow, Glasgow G12 8QQ, Scotland, UK. Telephone: ++ 141 330 4499 Fax: ++ 141 330 4100
E-mail: N.Spurway@bio.gla.ac.uk

About the Editors

Gisela Sjøgaard is Professor in Sports and Health Sciences at University of Southern Denmark, Odense. She earned her Ph.D. in muscle physiology at the Faculty of Natural Science and her Dr.Med.Sc. at the Faculty of Medicine at the University of Copenhagen. She recieved a University Gold Medal Award. She was the head of the department of physiology at the National Institute of Occupational Health in Denmark. She is member of a number of international committees in the area of sports and health sciences and editor as well referee of several scientific journals. Her main field of competence is human exercise physiology with focus on muscle mechanics, metabolism and fatigue. Sailing is her favorite sport for competition and leisure pleasure.

Jens Bangsbo is Associate Professor at the Institute of Exercise and Sport Sciences, University of Copenhagen, where he achieved his doctoral degree with the thesis „Physiology of Soccer – with a special reference to high intensity intermittent exercise". He has written more than one hundred original papers and reviews. He is the author of 12 books published in a number of different languages. He has received the „Biochemistry of Exercise" award. He is a member of the International Steering Group on Science and Football. He is a former professional soccer player and has played more than four hundred matches in the Danish top league as well as several matches in the Danish National team.

About the Authors

Finn Bojsen-Møller is Associated Professor, Laboratory for Functional Anatomy and Biomechanics, University of Copenhagen, Denmark. He is section editor of Acta Anatomica and Scandinavian Journal of Medicine and Science in Sports. He is member of the editorial board for several journals and he is member of the board of the Nordic Network for Research Physiotherapists. He is author of a great number of articles within sport medicine and functional anatomy as well as material properties of biological tissues.

Ole Crumlin-Pedersen is currently Director of the Centre for Maritime Archaeology of the National Museum of Denmark and Honorary Professor at the Institute of Medieval Archaeology at the Aarhus University. Since graduating as a Naval Architect he has been Head of the Viking Ship Museum in Roskilde and the Institute of Maritime Archaeology of the National Museum. He has conducted several excavation campaigns on Viking-Age and medieval ships in Denmark, Germany and Sweden, and written numerous articles and books on the early history of shipbuilding and on maritime aspects of Iron-Age and medieval cultural history.

Antonio Dal Monte is Professor at the Istituto di Scienza dello Sport, Dipartimento di Fisiologia e Biomeccanica, Rome, Italy. He is Scientific Director of Institute of Sport Science and head of the Department of Physiology and Biomechanics, Comitato Olimpico Nazionale Italiano – CONI (Italian National Olympics Committee). He has carried out research in evaluations of athletes and in biometrics in sport. He is the innovator of numerous ergometric instruments for application in his field of study. He has published more than 400 reviews, 10 books and various monographs. He is the president of the medical commissions of Italian track and field Federation; Italian Rowing Federation; Aero Club d'Italia and C.O.N.I.-C.N.R. He has been awarded Gold Star for Sport Merit and a honorary degree of the Ukrainian State University.

Leif Hambræus is Professor of Human Nutrition at the Faculty of Medicine, Uppsala University, Department of Medical Sciences, Nutrition. He certified as MD and received his Dr of Med Sci degree at the Faculty of Medicine, Karolinska Institute, Stockholm. He is scientific advisor in nutrition to the Swedish Olympic Committee and has personal experience from participating in several offshore sailing races in the Baltic. Professor Hambræus is the author of more than 350 scientific articles and reviews and editor/co-editor of several books. In recent years he has built up a metabolic unit for studies on energy and protein interaction in healthy adults as well as the effect of physical exercise on substrate utilization.

Heinemann, Klaus is Professor of sociology at the University of Hamburg. He has a Ph.D. in sociology at the Technische Hochschule Karlsruhe. His research emphases are sociology of economy and organisations, sociology and economy of sport and methods of empirical research. He has written 26 books and more than 150 articles. He was chair of the Scientific Advisory Board of the German Sport Federation from 1978 to 1990. He was editor of the „International Review for the Sociology of Sport" from 1988 to 1996.

Marco Marchetti is Professor of Human Physiology at Rome University „La Sapienza". He is Director of the Institute of Human Physiology and Director of postgraduate School in Sport Medicine at the same University. His main scientific interests are exercise and sport physiology and motor rehabilitation. Marchetti is a member of the Italian Sailing Federation.

Neil Spurway is Professor of Exercise Physiology in the Centre for Exercise Science and Medicine, University of Glasgow, Scotland. He got his first boat in 1948, has raced to national level in about a dozen dinghy classes since and is still active. From 1987-1994 he coached the Scottish Under 16 Sailing Squad. He is a member of the British Olympic Association's Exercise Physiology Steering Group, and has chaired the Physiology Section of the British Association of Sport and Exercise Sciences. His scientific work began in membrane biophysics, then moved upward through comparative muscle histochemistry and the physiology of blood vessels to studies of fatigue and training.

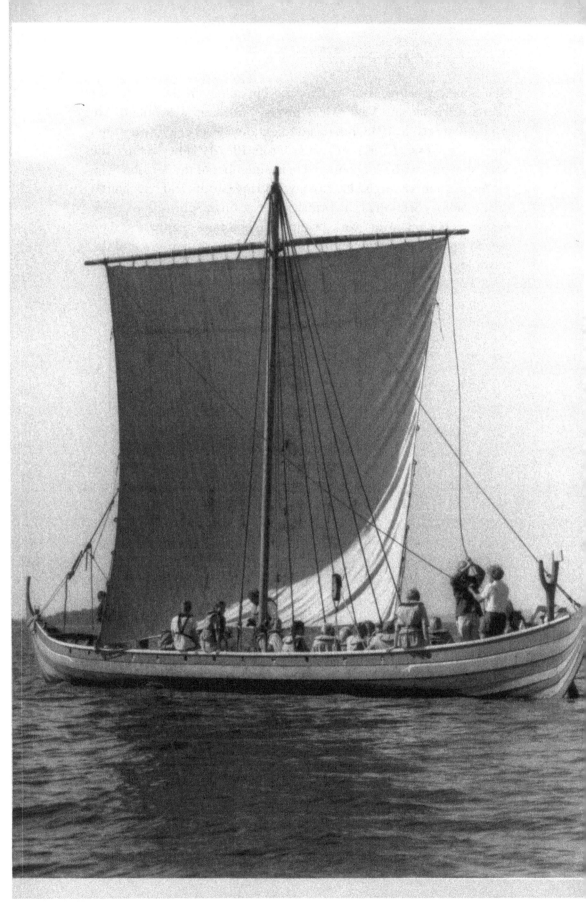

THE SPORTING ELEMENT IN VIKING SHIPS AND OTHER EARLY BOATS

Ole Crumlin-Pedersen

Synopsis

The paper presents some of the observations about the sporting element in early boats from Scandinavia that may be derived from written sources and archaeological finds. A competitive team-spirit very similar to that of modern sports teams was found among the young warriors in the halls of the chieftains and at the king's court. They would man fast and slender vessels, propelled by paddlers in the centuries BC, by oarsmen up to the 6th-7th centuries AD and at a later date by a combination of oarsmen and sail. By carefully studying the Viking-Age and older ship- and boatfinds we may find inspiration in constructional details that can be of interest to designers of modern boats for teams of paddlers or rowers, or for sailing.

When studying the ancient history of sport, we have to work from the combined evidence of archaeological finds, written sources and ancient pictures. In this way much information about the sporting elements in the culture of classical Greece has been extracted, since sport is described by ancient authors and depicted on vases, as well as indicated in excavations of arenas. As is well known, modern sport with the Olympic Games, marathon races etc. owes much to this classical heritage from Greece.

The question for us to investigate here is whether there was a similar situation among the Vikings and their ancestors in the North a thousand years and more ago. Even here we have some evidence of the same nature, a few written sources and pictures and a considerable quantity of archaeological finds.

My special field of study is the development of the ships and boats of Iron-Age and medieval Scandinavia. Here it is an interesting question whether the changes over time in the construction of ships should be attributed to purely functional demands, or whether other factors, including a sporting element, have influenced the designs in various phases.

To investigate this question it is necessary first of all to look for traces of sportsmanship in the written evidence. Our first problem, then, will be to define the term sport and to specify a general set of criteria that may characterize the term 'sport' in Viking-Age Scandinavia a millennium ago as well as today.

In continuation I shall use the term *sport* to describe *a physical leisure activity carried out to train skills, to improve health and/or to socialize individuals, combined with a competitive element for fun, for prestige and/or for materialistic reasons.* Several such activities are part of normal work situations or military training as well, however, so the problem remains how to identify the leisure element in the activity.

This is not easy for cultures without a distinct division between working hours and time spent on other activities in society. Besides, the nature of sporting activities changes over time. In different cultures and cultural phases, different types of sport are prevalent, and *changes* in the form and function of sport occur precisely in phases when there are paradigmatic changes (11). We cannot therefore blindly apply more recent standards for *sport* to the situation a thousand years ago without the risk of missing the point.

It is against this background that I shall look at one of the potential sources for the study of Viking society: the medieval sagas of the North, employing a critical approach, since they were written down centuries later than the events they describe, and under Christian influence. In the *Edda* of the Icelandic scholar Snorri Sturluson, written around 1220 AD, we learn about *Valhalla* as a pre-Christian paradise for the Viking warriors who died on the battlefield (14). In Valhalla the warriors had a great time fighting all day long and being restored to life in the evening so that they could feast with their god Odin, and the next morning begin fighting anew. You just need to replace the battlefield by a modern sportsground with teams playing hockey or football to see that this model might also be considered as paradise by many of the sports-teams of today.

This story might be taken as proof of the strong sporting spirit of the Vikings. There are indications in other sources, however, that Snorri based this narrative on two different ancient myths (8). The first is the myth of a life after death as a guest of Odin, offered to members of those noble families which were thought to be the descendants of the god. The other myth is that of a continuous battle taking place in the cold and grey underworld between two parties, never to be ended so that the deceased warriors could go to rest. If this is right, there is no true support for joyful Viking sportsmanship in the myths underlying the Valhalla story.

There are other sources, however, which reflect a spirit of sportsmanship in training young men of the 10th-11th centuries in body and mind to be excellent swordsmen, horsemen or sailors. In the continuation I shall concentrate on evidence reflecting what we may term *a boat-racing spirit.*

The old scaldic verses sometimes in a quick glimpse reflect pride in swift sailing, as in a poem in the saga of Grettir, relating to his forefather Ønund, who had lost one leg in battle and later plied the Atlantic in a heavy deep-sea cargo-carrier (9):

> *Once Wooden-Leg was one among heroes*
> *when he raced ahead in his swift vessel*
> *in a cool sword-attack.*
> *Now, fed up with life, a miserable One-leg*
> *is chugging along towards Iceland*
> *in his deep-sea tramp.*

This is a good specification of some of those parameters which characterize Viking heroes:

> *they are young,*
> *they sail in a fast ship,*
> *they display bravery in action and good swordsmanship.*

To judge from this and other scaldic verses of the 10th and 11th centuries, this ideology was prevalent among the warriors at the king's court. A king or petty king would surround himself with a group of personal warriors, large or small, for safety reasons but also as a symbol of his high status. In order to display his power and prestige, the king would present to his faithful men and allies high status gifts in gold or of exquisite craftsmanship. In order to assemble the necessary riches to be able to win fame as a generous king, he had to raid foreign coasts for their wealth, which would subsequently be distributed in part to his followers.

Thus in pre-Christian Nordic Viking society there were, beside the large majority of the population peacefully tilling their fields, small groups of young men, eager to win fame and wealth as the warriors of a famous chieftain or king. In these groups there was a constant spirit of sportsmanship in the attempt to be the best man to handle a sword, a horse or a ship. The king or chieftain was in the position to provide for the construction of the best and fastest ships, and there was a steady impetus to develop these even further in order for them to be superior to those of one's opponents (Fig. 1). This competitive spirit has much in common with that of modern professional sports teams.

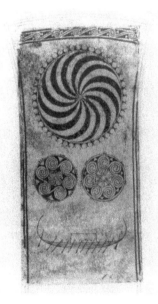
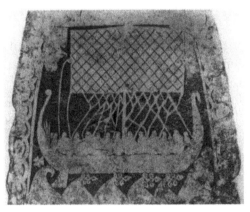

Fig. 1 Ships from Gotland picture-stones. Left: rowing vessel from Bro, 5th-6th century AD. Right: Sailing vessel from Hejnum Riddare, 8th century AD. From Sune Lindqvist: Gotlands Bildsteine. Stockholm 1941.

Whether or not we can call this range of activities 'sport', the effect of this social mechanism was the development of vessels for war (and cultic use) that were highly sophisticated in their design and lines; so much so that we may even today gain new insight from them in optimizing vessels for paddling, rowing and sailing. In fact, in Bronze-Age and Iron-Age Scandinavia shipbuilding started with the development of such high-status vessels for warriors to paddle or row, and it was not until the middle of the first millenium AD that the sail was introduced and even later that ordinary cargo-carrying ships were built in the North (5).

The reason for this late development of sailing vessels in Scandinavia probably lay in the fact that chieftains needed a considerable number of followers for security and for displaying their prestige when travelling to religious or secular gatherings. Such journeys were almost exclusively made by boat, and here the chieftain would have a full crew to man the paddles or oars. This was a more stable means of propulsion than the wind, which might fade away for days on end or blow from the wrong direction. This led to the development of slender, light-weight vessels that could be beached and re-launched easily by the crew alone. With the addition of the sail to ships of this nature the basis for long-range raids was established, with the 'hit-and-run tactics' used by the Vikings in their attacks on England and France in the 9th century.

Thus the beginning of the story of shipbuilding in the North was *not* that of an initial stage with robust cargo-carriers, later to be refined into more elegant ships. On the contrary, the earliest Iron-Age and Viking-Age ships known to us are the most exquisite examples of sophisticated craftsmanship – at the cutting edge of the technology available at the time.

Today the study of these vessels offers us a perspective on the current experience with paddled, rowed or sail-carrying boats used for sports. We may even find ourselves in a position where these old boat-types inspire modern man to design new boat-types for leisure activities, especially for long-range cruising and team-racing – because that was exactly what these ancient boats were built for.

The earliest evidence for such vessels, manned with large crews of paddlers, is to be found on the Bronze-Age rock carvings of Scandinavia, as well as engraved on bronze objects of that period (10). The ships are shown with a peculiar shape with beaks projecting out from both ends. At an early stage of research several attempts were made to interpret these as skinboats, floats or even sledges.

In 1921, however, excavations in a small bog at Hjortspring in southern Denmark brought to light the remains of an approx. 19 m long boat for 20 paddlers, shaped exactly as those in the pictures and deposited here with the weapons and gear of a full team of warriors (Fig. 2). Evidently the local population had been able to resist a seaborne attack around 325 BC and had handed over the ship and equipment

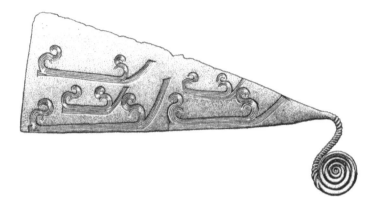

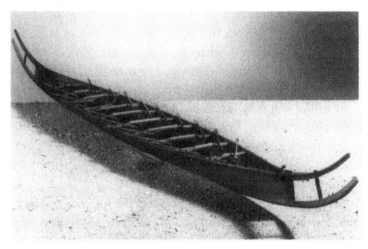

Fig. 2 Engraving of ships on a Bronze-Age razor from Solbjerg, 6th-7th century BC, and model of the 4th century BC Hjortspring boat. From Flemming Kaul: Ships on Bronzes. *Copenhagen 1998, and same:* Bronzealderens både. *Roskilde 1998.*

of the defeated group as a war-booty offering to the gods. After difficult conservation- and restoration-work the find is now exhibited at the National Museum in Copenhagen (13).

The Hjortspring boat is 'primitive' only in the sense that it is not metal-fastened. All parts are assembled with a sewing technique using thin cords embedded in a resin. But this technique, in combination with sophisticated craftsmanship in the woodwork, produced a vessel which was extraordinarily light and resiliant. The seats for the paddlers are part of a framing system with lashed frames, and these as well as other details display features that are highly functional and esthetically pleasing. A replica of this boat is at present under construction near the finding place, and the members of the building team, including several engineers and computer experts, are deeply fascinated by the exceptional standard of the original vessel, to which they are striving to live up. The boat will be launched in 1999 to be taken on extensive trials.

There is no point in suggesting that the Hjortspring boat should serve as a prototype for a new, modern class of paddled sports-boats for team-racing, as it is simply too complex a design for that. There may, however, be a lesson to be learnt from the trials as to the paddling technique and other features which at the time of construction of the original boat had been practised in the North over a period of at least 1,500 years – and no doubt in a strongly competitive spirit, which produced the Hjortspring boat as the ultimate design of that period in fast and light paddled boats.

If we jump six centuries forward in time, we find the first boats propelled by oars. At that time, in the centuries after the birth of Christ, the influence of Roman technology was strong, even outside the Roman empire. Elements of maritime technology were picked up by warriors from the North serving in the Roman army and navy and brought back home to be absorbed or rejected as inspiration for the construction and propulsion of local warships (5) (Figs. 3-4). The Nydam ship from

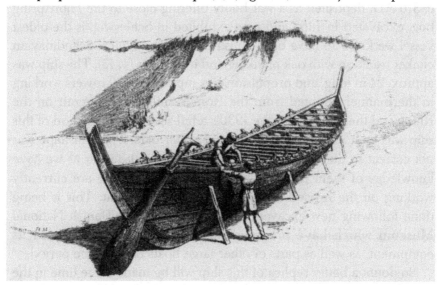

Fig. 3 The Nydam ship drawn up on the beach. Reconstruction drawing by Magnus Petersen 1897.

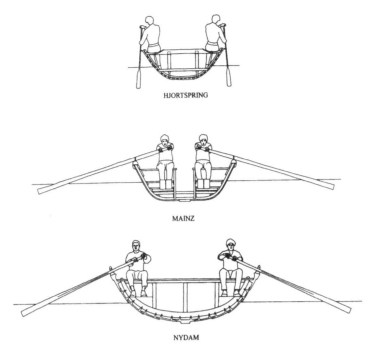

Fig. 4 Cross-sections of the vessels from Hjortspring (4th century BC), Mainz A (c. 400 AD) and Nydam (c. 330 AD), showing the system of propulsion by paddling or rowing. After Crumlin-Pedersen 1997a.

c. 310 AD, deposited as a war-booty offering close to the Hjortspring bog, excavated in 1863 and now exhibited in Schleswig, is the oldest vessel we know to have been constructed in the typical Scandinavian clinker tradition with oak planking and iron rivets (4, 13). The ship was approx. 24 m long, and propulsion was supplied by 30 rowers working in the manner adopted from the Roman military river-craft on the Rhine and the Danube. In the 1930's a full-scale reconstruction of this ship was built in Germany and tested under oars. The hullshape was not correct so that the experience from these trials, as far as we have knowledge of them today, is of little value for us. We are currently working on the revised drawings of the original boat. This is being done following new excavations in the bog by the Danish National Museum which have provided further parts of the boat and its equipment, as well as parts of other large boats of the same period.

No doubt a better replica of this ship will be made some time in the near future, and with this vessel extensive trials should be undertaken to study the way in which such a large rowing-boat reacts under various conditions. This might yield new evidence about the principles of long-range cruising with large rowing teams, and it would be natural to undertake such trials in cooperation with people actively engaged in the design of various types of modern rowed vessels for sport.

If we jump another six centuries ahead in time, we arrive in the middle of the Viking Age, at a time when sail propulsion had been fully integrated in the maritime technology of the North, yet without losing contact with the experience of propulsion by rowing. At this time, in the 10th and 11th centuries AD, the first vessels built especially for cargo-carrying appear among the finds. They were relatively broad and deep, with proportions similar to those of the classical Viking vessel excavated in 1880 in a burial mound at Gokstad in Norway where the length of 24 m is 4.7 times the width (12).

Finds of warships from the area of Viking-Age Denmark, however, are quite different in their construction and proportions from those of the Gokstad ship and the cargo-carriers (Fig. 5). They are real longships,

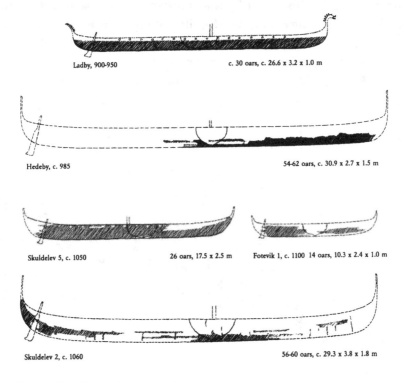

Ladby, 900-950   c. 30 oars, c. 26.6 x 3.2 x 1.0 m

Hedeby, c. 985   54-62 oars, c. 30.9 x 2.7 x 1.5 m

Skuldelev 5, c. 1050   26 oars, 17.5 x 2.5 m   Fotevik 1, c. 1100 14 oars, 10.3 x 2.4 x 1.0 m

Skuldelev 2, c. 1060   56-60 oars, c. 29.3 x 3.8 x 1.8 m

Fig. 5 Warships of the 10th and 11th centuries drawn to the same scale with an indication by shading of the recorded/preserved parts of the vessels. The cross-sections are indicated amidships. After Crumlin-Pedersen 1997a.

27

the lengths of which are from six up to eleven times as much as the width. Such ships have been found in burial mounds at Hedeby and Ladby, as well as on the sea-bed at Hedeby, Skuldelev, Roskilde and Fotevik. They give us detailed insight into shipbuilding technology, as well as into the different standards of craftsmanship applied in the construction of ships in accordance with the symbolic role of the ship. Thus there is a distinct difference between those low-status ships that were built by the local farming communities at the king's command - using recycled wood and patchwork repairs, as in the Skuldelev 5-ship (3) – and the high-status royal ships built with sophisticated craftsmanship and from timber of excellent quality, as in the Hedeby 1-ship.

The latter ship-type is probably the one known from contemporary scaldic poetry under the term *skeið*, especially applied by Norwegian poets to the long Danish warships with their flexible sides. The Hedeby longship of this type was originally about 30 m long and only 2.7 m wide, yet equipped for sail as well as for about 60 oars (6) (Fig. 6). Racing along in this ship of royal standard under oars or sail must have been a sporting experience for life for anyone who had the opportunity to try, bringing the poem about Ønund One-leg to mind:

> *Once Wooden-Leg was one among heroes*
> *when he raced ahead in his swift vessel in a cool sword-attack.*

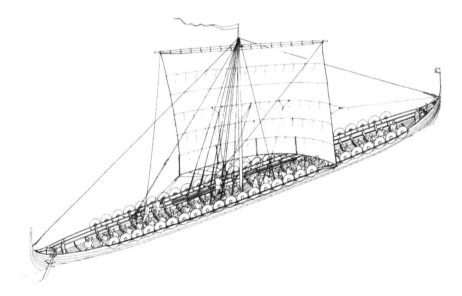

Fig. 6 Artist's impression of the longship Hedeby 1 under sail. After Crumlin-Pedersen 1997b.

The word *skeið*, by the way, is related to an Indo-European verb meaning 'to cleave', bringing another fast ship-type of a much later period, the *clipper*, to mind as a parallel. In both cases the ships were extraordinarily fast by the standards of their time, and they are characterized by a designation relating to their fast passage through the waves. With the tea-clippers of 19th century there was such strong competition to be the first to bring the new harvest of tea to the market in London that bets were placed, as if the ships were taking part in a horse-race.

No full-scale working reconstruction has yet been built of the Hedeby longship and it will indeed be a difficult task to do so, as the planking was originally made up of thin oak-planks of superior quality, several of which were over 10 m in length. The details of the structure were executed to the highest standards in order to combine strength and light weight. The original ship would have been a true racer, constructed to cut its way through the waves in an 'organic' way, not unlike fish and sea-mammals that constantly adjust their shape to minimize their resistance, though for the ship with much more limited movements, preliminary torsional, and well controlled in the structural lay-out of the vessel.

The same principles of lightness of weight and flexibility of the hull are found in the other warships known to us, though not to the same high standard as in the Hedeby longship. The contrast to the 17m-long Skuldelev 5-ship for 26 oars is especially marked, as this ship was built from recycled wood and repaired over and over again to a point where it was hardly seaworthy (3). From 12th-century written sources we know that the king ordered each district in the country to build and man ships for coastal defence, and that fines had to be paid if each individual farmer did not deliver his share of the construction materials. When such a ship was old and needed replacement in the opinion of the royal controller, while the locals found it good enough for a few more seasons, a test had to be carried out: If the ship could manage under sail in open waters with no more than one man bailing, the ship was declared seaworthy. This is exactly the type of ship that we have found in the Skuldelev 5-ship, of which a full-scale working reconstruction (Fig. 7) has been built in Roskilde west of Copenhagen, where the original Skuldelev Viking ships are on display at the Viking Ship Museum.

This reconstruction, the 'Helge Ask', as well as the 'Roar Ege', replicating the Skuldelev 3-ship, a small coaster, and 'Saga Siglar', built

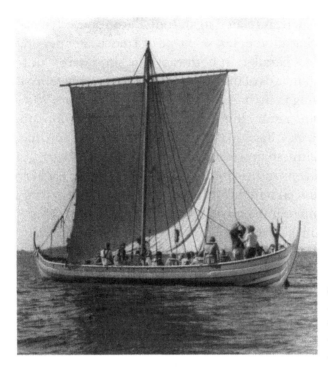

Fig. 7 The Skuldelev
5 replica Helge Ask
on the Roskilde Fjord.
Photo Viking Ship
Museum, Roskilde.

as a copy of Skuldelev 1, the deep-sea trader, have given us valuable practical experience with the various ship-types of the 11th century. For all ships resilience is the keyword. The hulls are not constructed with a rigid structure but with slender resilient elements to absorb the strains of the waves in the open sea. At the same time this feature enables the ships to maintain a steady speed in tacking against the waves without the hull being braked by slamming.

In the underwater hull of the deep-sea trader Skuldelev 1 the cross-section shows an anomaly in the fair run of the lines that could be characterized as a 'negative keel' at both sides of the proper keel (Fig. 8). This feature no doubt served to steady the course under sail. At the same time, air is drawn down in a spiral along these lines underneath the ship. The original reason for this peculiarity is not known in detail but according to our observations, it may have served as an air-cushion

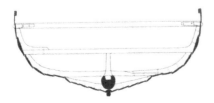

Fig. 8 Cross-section of the Skuldelev 1
cargo-ship, showing the 'negative keel'
formed by the inclined angle of the fifth
strake from the keel.

in the bow to dampen slamming and at the same time the vortex of air under the ship may have reduced the friction of the hull by lubricating part of the planking.

The Viking ships were steered with spade-rudders placed aft on the starboard side, named from this feature. In the Mediterranean the ships were fitted with a rudder on each side aft to maintain a steady course under sail. With only one rudder there would be increased resistance at the starboard side of the ship in relation to that at the port side, and the ship would tend to turn to starboard if not counteracted by the rudder. To compensate for this, the Vikings in some cases deliberately gave the blade of the rudder a hydrofoil shape. This is strikingly demonstrated by a rudder found at Vorså in the Kattegat (2) (Fig. 9). Here the greater part of the blade is asymmetrical in such a way that the flow around the rudder when sailing will give a 'lift', providing a moment that counteracts the effect of the friction of the rudder. This effect has been noticed in practical experiments with copies of this rudder on some of our reconstructed ships.

The Vorså rudder also gave rise to other interesting observations. In one case a new rudder was made considerably thicker than the original one for safety reasons – with the unexpected result that the rudder broke when the ship was sailing in a strong wind abeam with high waves. The ship tended to slide sidewards down from the crest of the highest waves, and under such conditions the new rudder was too stiff, resulting in a fracture. Under similar conditions the original rudder would have bent sidewards and thus have absorbed the tension. This is a good example of the importance of flexibility in the design of these ships.

There was even more to be learned from this rudder for the careful observer and experimental archaeologist. We were astonished by the fact that the aft edge of a rudder of such a fine hydrofoil shape was cut off abruptly and that the rudder ended with a small heel at the lower end. In action, however, we noticed that a steady flow of air was drawn in a spiral along the after edge and released at the heel. This worked perfectly and prevented the rudder from vibrating when the ship was sailing at high speed. It may also have an effect in providing an addition to the rudder-area without an increase in the wet surface of the rudder. On one occation the heel broke off the rudder of one of our ships and immediately the rudder started to react by vibrating because of the lack of a stable flow of air.

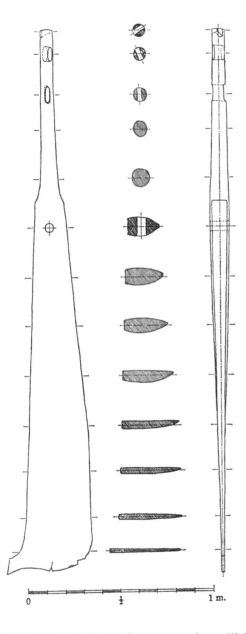

Fig. 9 The Viking-Age side-rudder from Vorså, Denmark. After Crumlin-Pedersen 1966.

I hope that these few examples will have served to indicate that there is a lesson to be learned from these early boats, not only for archaeologists but also for naval architects and others interested in the development of modern vessels for sporting activities on the water. At the Centre for Maritime Archaeology, established by the Danish National Research Foundation and the National Museum, we are currently engaged in investigating these ships in cooperation with naval architect

Leif Wagner Smitt of the Danish Maritime Institute. The results of extensive trials with these working reconstructions have been published in Danish (1) and in the near future they will be compared with data from tank tests and calculations and published in English (7). Here we have a unique opportunity to establish a bridge between the past and the present and to bring forgotten knowledge about important naval architectural aspects back to life, to be utilized in the construction of modern boats.

References

1. Andersen, E. & al. *Roar Ege – Skuldelev 3 skibet som arkæologisk eksperiment.* Roskilde 1997.
2. Crumlin-Pedersen, O. Two Danish Side Rudders. *The Mariner's Mirror* 52, 3, pp. 251-261, 1966.
3. Crumlin-Pedersen, O. Gensyn med Skuldelev 5 – et ledingsskib? *Festskrift til Olaf Olsen*, pp. 137-156. København 1988.
4. Crumlin-Pedersen, O. The boats and ships of the Angles and Jutes. In S. McGrail (ed.): *Maritime Celts, Frisians and Saxons.* CBA Research Report 71, pp. 98-116. London 1990.
5. Crumlin-Pedersen, O. Large and small warships of the North. In A.N. Jørgensen & B.L.Clausen (eds.): *Military Aspects of Scandinavian Society in a European Perspective, AD 1-1300.* PNM Studies in Archaeology & History 2, pp. 184-194. Copenhagen 1997a.
6. Crumlin-Pedersen, O. *Viking-Age ships and shipbuilding in Hedeby/Haithabu and Schleswig.* Ships & Boats of the North 2. Roskilde 1997b.
7. Crumlin-Pedersen, O. & O. Olsen (eds.), forthcoming: *The Skuldelev Ships.* Ships & Boats of the North 4. Roskilde.
8. Davidson, H.R.E. *Gods and Myths of Northern Europe.* London. (The Realm of Odin, pp. 149-153) 1964.
9. Gunnarsson, G. *Sagaen om Gretter den Stærke.* København (p. 11, translation by the author) 1968.
10. Kaul, F. Ships on Bronzes. In O. Crumlin-Pedersen & B.M.Thye (eds.): *The Ship as Symbol in Prehistoric and Medieval Scandinavia.* PNM Studies in Archaeology & History 1, pp. 59-70. Copenhagen 1995.
11. Krogsgaard, O. Idræt. In E. Alstrup & P.E. Olsen (eds.) *Dansk kulturhistorisk Opslagsværk*, pp. 378-381. København 1991.
12. Nicolaysen, N. *Langskibet fra Gokstad ved Sandefjord - The Viking-Ship discovered at Gokstad in Norway.* Kristiania 1882.
13. Rieck, F. & O. Crumlin-Pedersen *Både fra Danmarks Oldtid.* Roskilde. (Hjortspring, pp. 55-74) 1988.
14. Simek, R. *Lexikon der germanischen Mythologie.* Stuttgart (Snorra Edda, pp. 366-367; Walhall, pp. 454-456) 1984.

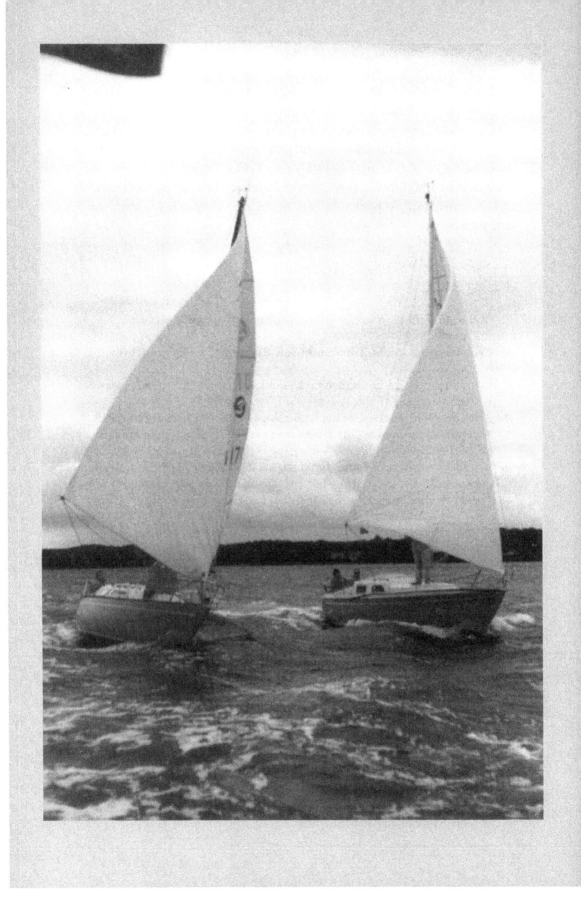

Boat construction
– drag and aerodynamics

Antonio Dal Monte, Claudio Gallozzi & Dario Dalla Vedova

Synopsis

*Sailing is the result of a complex combination of physical pheno-
mena closely interrelated. More, the regatta rules and the continuous
evolution offered by new materials, new design and construction
techniques and simulation software continue to add new variables to the problem. The authors shortly examine the modern boats,
foils, sails, the materials they are made of and what keeps up our
interest in studying an art as old as sailing.*

Introduction

Sailing is the result of a complex combination of physical phenomena,
many of which do not spring naturally to mind (3, 4). Think, for
example, about the dynamics of sailing against the wind, or about the
fact that some craft can travel faster than the wind acting on them.
This is made possible by exploiting the peculiarities of the sailing zone:
the place where air and water meet, that is to say the system of two
fluids in relative reciprocal movement having very different physical
properties and behaviour.

More, the aerodynamic and hydrodynamic phenomena governing
the art of sailing are closely interrelated, and it is very often difficult, if
not impossible, to pinpoint the cause producing a given effect (1). It is
difficult to find the exact parameter on which to act and to come up
with a physical-mathematical theory that can successfully and reliably

simulate real conditions. It is a mistake, for instance, to study the form of sailing equipments without taking into account the type of craft it will be installed on. Neither is it possible to design sails and foils in accordance with aerodynamic theory alone without taking into account the construction constraints imposed by available technologies and materials.

This is clearly demonstrated by the history of sailboats, sailing technology and the development of the principal trading routes. In ancient times, ships transporting goods needed to have considerable cargo capacities, therefore wide hulls with little ballast and draught. It was for this reason that they had square sails fixed onto a number of masts, and round keels. They could not therefore haul to windward, and could not sail before the wind, otherwise the fore sails would be spilled, but had to maintain a tack varying from athwart to slack, almost always wearing. For this reason, the Ocean routes were for centuries those going along the Trades, thus reducing the occasions where head winds would occur.

The growth of the Indies market and more intense relations with Australia brought with it the search for faster craft that could also haul upon the wind. This led to the study and construction of clippers, with their efficient equipment. These vessels, having a smaller cargo capacity than traditional sailing ships and being more difficult to handle, were also much faster and able to compete with the new steamships, in relation to which they could still ensure cost savings. Changes to installed equipment produced significant changes in tacks and consequently in practicable routes.

Moving on to more recent times, the evolution of the shape of hulls and sails has been enormously influenced by the use of craft for sporting purposes, and consequently by rating and regatta rules.

Regatta Rules

When sailing races began in the last century, the need quickly emerged to set forth and standardise regatta rules for competition routes and craft used. This led to the creation of "Class" associations in charge of arranging races among similar craft adhering to a set of rules for that particular class. One-design regattas are still commonplace today. The sport of sailing is indeed represented in the Olympic Games by one-design races. It is interesting to note on this point that the most recent of classes is Laser, designed in 1971, while the Star, introduced in 1911 and updated over the years, is still extremely valid from technical and competitive viewpoints.

But of one-design racing, the rules have played and continue to play a major role in the development of craft. One of the most evident examples of this are the rating rules set to allow comparisons between craft performance thus permitting craft of different sizes and construction to compete with one another. It is well-known for example that the speed of a boat chiefly depends on the length of the waterline, its weight, surface area of its sails and other variables. Rating formulas can be used to assign to each factor a relative weight in order to establish, for each single craft, a rating that can be used to adjust the time taken to complete the regatta course. One of the rating rules that had the greatest influence on the design of sailing boats was the I.O.R., adopted in 1970.

For this type of rating, some measurements to determine the rating were made at given points of the keel. This caused designers to force the boat forms in order to obtain the best possible rating result, creating hulls with non-conventional forms at the points where measurements were taken, resulting in inefficiency in the water. The rating also adversely affected weight stability and wetted surface (and consequently the shape stability), so that crafts were generally not as stable as they could have been.

Notwithstanding this, the construction philosophy inspired by the I.O.R. reigned for many years, and not only in racing boats. It was only replaced by a new rating system at the end of the 1970s: the I.M.S. (International Measurement System).

The I.M.S. was a revolution for rating systems since, for the first time, powerful simulation software could be used to define a craft's characteristics. The I.M.S. was borne in the 1970s at the M.I.T. (Massachusetts Institute of Technology), being a research to simulate the performance of various types of sailboats using computer software. This objective was pursued by using the enormous database of aerodynamic and hydrodynamic data obtained from wind tunnel and water flume studies. This data, entered in the system of physical equations governing sailing, was used to supply the maximum theoretical speed that each craft could reach.

With the modern I.M.S. system, a software called Line Processing Program (L.P.P.) contains water flume data that is used in conjunction with the output from a tool called "hull-scanner", which in turn is used to create a virtual 3D model of the keels of various craft. Data gathered, plus accurate measurements of sails, equipment, weights and static righting moments, are entered in a second software program called Velocity Prediction Program (V.P.P.) which, performing some loops, comes up with an ideal state of equilibrium for the system of aero-hydrodynamic forces. From a physical viewpoint, the equilibrium of forces means that the maximum theoretical speed in a stable condition has been reached, since the craft can no longer accelerate (without undergoing a predominance of propulsive forces) nor slow down (predominance of drag elements). As the forces acting on the keel and on the sails constitute the square of water and air speeds respectively, it is possible to identify the maximum achievable speed for each configuration of a particular type of craft. The procedure is repeated for the various wind speeds and for all the tacks that the craft assumes. In this way, it is possible to have the vessel's global theoretical performance.

Since the I.M.S. makes it possible to predict the performance of all sailboat types and consequently to reward or penalise craft, the study of craft equipment was resumed with new vigour upon the introduction of the new measuring system. Much longer rudders and keels appeared to raise hydrodynamic efficiency, and there was a return of vertical bows to maximise waterline length. This led to faster I.M.S.-designed craft than those designed for the I.O.R., since the new system involves very accurate keel measurements, obviating the need for special shapes adopted previously.

Aero-hydrodynamics

In this continuous search for better performance, the study of fluid-dynamic aspects of the keel, foils and sails clearly takes on considerable importance. Logically, the lower resistance encountered by a body moving in a fluid or system of fluids, the higher the maximum achievable speed will be. This is why the reduction in the "drag" of the keel or the optimisation of the sail shape are the principal factors a designer can work on to enhance a vessel's performance (4, 6, 8).

Although the laws of fluid statics and fluid mechanics have been applied for thousands of years, their physical formulation goes back to the 17th and 18th centuries. Scientific studies conducted using instruments such as the wind tunnel and water flume began at the beginning of this century. The correct methodological and scientific study of such an established practice therefore started in relatively recent times. Below are brief descriptions of the guidelines followed by modern designers in designing and constructing sailboats. To simplify matters, hydrodynamic (keels and foils) and aerodynamic research will be dealt with in two separate paragraphs.

Keels and foils

The earliest sailors noticed that boats, moving through the water, came up against considerable resistance. This is due to the fact that, in order to move, the hull must displace great quantities of water, generating waves and wake, that is to say dispersive phenomena responsible for significant induced drag (4, 6). In later times, mathematical formula was drawn up for this type of problem. It was observed that every displacing vessel has a maximum theoretical speed (Vc) based on a series of constants (K) and the square root of the vessel's waterline length (L): $V_C = K \times \sqrt{L}$ (Fig. 1). This means that, all

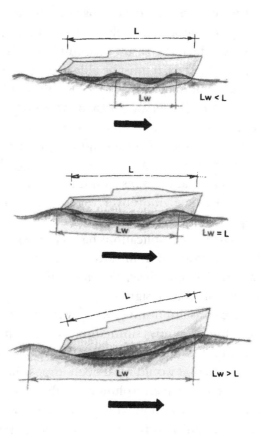

Fig. 1 The maximum theoretical speed for every displacing vessel has a maximum value depending on a series of constamts (K) and the square root of the vessel's waterline length (L): $V_C = K \times \sqrt{L}$

39

things being equal, the longer a boat, the faster it will be. Ancient peoples had actually grasped this principle, and craft such as the Egyptian felucca, Polynesian pirogue or Viking ship have been studied in depth in recent times. Nowadays, the techniques used to obtain high sailing speeds have developed along two paths: the study of lengthened shapes, leading to the advent of multihull craft and record-breaking boats, and the study of planar keels. In fact, the other way of overcoming the "barrier" represented by the waves is that of moving at a speed at which the boat is no longer against the wave, but receives from the water a hydrodynamic support such as to lift over the water. Although this alternative has many limits and difficulties, it is still the only way for traditional sailboats. This does not mean however the end of the study and design of keels after a thousand years evolution. A vessel's keel is indeed the result of a number of compromises coming from a variety of needs. It must be able to ensure suitable dimensions (=cargo capacity), the stability of form, the minimum drag and wetted surface, the offsetting of leeway and a number of dynamic properties in response to transitory phenomena such as waves and gusts of wind. It must at the same time be lightweight, while remaining suitably rigid and structurally resistant. It must accordingly have the least possible ballast located at its lowest point in order to obtain a high righting moment. The keel, moreover, together with its foils, must provide a lift to oppose that generated by the wind on the sails in order to limit leeway (6). Further complications have been added, as mentioned previously, by the introduction of rating and racing rules which, by establishing measuring penalties and competition courses, have had a significant impact on boat design.

The constant honing of study instruments, such as the water flume and fluid dynamics simulation software, has made it possible to carry out rapid and (often) cost-saving experiments on a variety of new solutions that would have been impossible just a few years ago. Simulation software has revolutionised the waterlines of modern racing keels and, indirectly, of all craft, since they make it possible to evaluate in theory a hull's performance, weighing up the effect of each single variable on the behaviour of the entire system. The result of this has been a radical change in waterlines, with the search for planar keels and the optimisation of all foils.

Foils have in a certain sense marked the steps of evolution of keels. The first one made from the round-keeled, stable vessels to the modern keel was when it first came into somebody's mind to haul to windward, and so to place in the water a surface that could offset leeway. The second fundamental step was that of putting as much weight as possible inside, or rather at the extremity of the foils in order to increase the righting moment without having to increase displacement. As can be imagined, each of these phases was not without difficulty from a design and technological viewpoint. In some cases, it was necessary to re-invent the construction method in order to obtain the desired results. Moving on to more modern times, the in-depth study of foils has chiefly been concerned with:

- hydrodynamic analysis and optimisation, with the study of elliptical sections, as these correspond better to the ideal lift distribution;
- the study of various types of "torpedoes" attached to the lower extremity of keels to concentrate ballast there and create winglet able to reduce induced drag;
- the application of moving parts and the study of tilting foils to try and optimise performance in the various operating configurations.

It should be added that in practice, the shape of the immersed part of the vessel is different from the design, producing greater drag owing to:

- more or less broad fluctuations caused by the pitch, leading to dispersive, periodical phenomena such as vortices;
- a greater parasitic drag owing to the topside;
- the possibility of cavitation phenomena affecting the two faces of the keel, since the windward face is close to the water surface when the boat is listing (heeling).

These are all factors that can be adjusted significantly in the design phase, and give an idea of the difficulties and complexity of this type of work.

Sails

To move through the water, sailboats use the aerodynamic propulsion generated by the interaction of the wind and the sails. That is why the "engine" of sailboats has always been carefully studied. This ongoing research is due to the fact that for practical, technological and construction reasons, the sails of a vessel are a strange aerodynamic thing (1, 2, 7). They cannot for example constitute rigid surfaces since they have to be quickly raised and lowered and, within certain limits, they must be adaptable to differing needs. The materials with which sails are made have continually been replaced by what new technologies have to offer. Technological progress, together with construction and regatta rules, have gone to establish the shape of sails up to the present day.

With reference to fluid-dynamics, sails may be seen as special wings (8). They work indeed in a three-dimensional aerodynamic field, and are heavily influenced by the interaction with all the boat's equipment, such as the mast, the rigging and above all the presence of other sails. This has made it extremely difficult to study and evaluate the aerodynamic validity of each single element, since it is not always possible to apply the law of overlapping effects. A system acting in such a complex way must indeed always be evaluated as a whole. Furthermore, the wind tunnel and modern simulation software often have significant limits when they are used to study such systems because, for a number of reasons, they are unable to correctly simulate dynamic phenomena such as the generation of lift or turbulence, especially in the presence of complex interactions.

The efficiency of a sail, for example, changes considerably according to the angle of inclination with respect to the water surface (2, 5, 6). This is because some air is deviated in a more or less turbulent manner, generating dispersion and considerable induced drag, and because of changes to the characteristic angles of attack of the profile.

The aerodynamic situation is further complicated by the boundary layer generated by the wind in proximity to the sea. As air is not an ideal fluid, its movement near any surface is slowed down by viscosity phenomena (vertical gradient), until it is stopped. This is particularly true for medium or slight breezes when viscous forces have the better of kinetic forces. More, the effects of the tridimensional aerodynamic field make both the wind direction and speed variable as one moves from the surface of the sea up to the mast/sail. This enforces considerable skills for the crew and sails designers and maker in order to obtain a perfect trim of the system.

In order to understand more fully the evolution of sail shapes, some historical and technological considerations are necessary at this point. As we saw in the introduction, the global shape of sailboats has changed greatly over the centuries according to the use made of vessels. Broadkeeled merchant shipping, for instance, could not keep a close-hauled tack, and so had square sails. This type of sail required special equipment and many sailors to handle it. These sails worked exclusively by generating wind resistance, and not lift, as is the case for modern sails. For this reason, and because they were used on merchant ships, the materials and cuts were selected according to their resistance, not their weight or efficiency. The appearance of the clipper and its commercial sails led to an increase in speed, but this was offset by the drop in cargo capacity. It led in any case to a significant technological change in the way sails were made. This change was indeed the prelude to a host of modern-day innovations, also due to the availability of new materials and to the transformation of sailing from a commercial activity to an hight level sport.

This change was clearly seen with the first America's Cup races held in the past century. The first rules established that challenging boats had to sail to the regatta in America by themselves, whichever part of the world they came from. It was very clear from the first few races that European boats, with their heavy sea-going equipment and sails that had crossed the Atlantic for the race would never be able to beat the fast, lightweight American craft expressly designed for that type of competition, and that would never have travelled beyond the calm waters of Newport.

In recent times, the availability of design software and of materials such as kevlar, mylar and carbon have repeatedly transformed the way of designing and constructing sails. These materials are lightweight, resistant and indeformable, until they eventually break. On the other hand, they require special, customised manufacturing. This has produced practically ideal shapes for profiles and extremely lightweight materials, although production costs are high and sails do not last so long.

Materials

This final paragraph is dedicated to a description of the principal features and applications of new materials. They have a great importance in the building of racing boat, sails and hulls and, as in other sports, have a significant impact on the way all modern boats are constructed (4, 7).

Historically, the first non-conventional material the boat designers were attracted from in the 1950s was plastic: a construction material as resistant as steel, as light as wood and imperishable. Its greatest quality however was seen to be its pliability, making it possible to shape objects very simply and quickly. The first fibreglass boats were produced in the 1960s. They were at first an alternative to traditional wooden constructions, before going on to gradually replace existing materials. The main advantages of fibreglass production were the lower costs and the possibility of mass-producing boats. Plastic too has evolved in recent decades. It is now more correct to talk of "composite materials" containing carbon and resins. Glass is now used with other materials such as kevlar and carbon, and there are various types of bonding agents (resins) such as polyester, vinyl and epoxy resin.

To understand the extraordinary growth of composite materials in modern times, we should briefly mention the principal requirements asked of materials for boat-building. A material must be resistant to complex three-dimensional stress, behave in a non-fragile manner and be as light as possible. Furthermore, it must be easy to shape in order

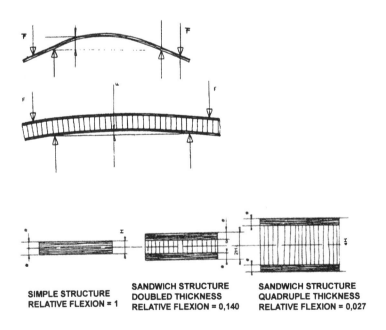

SIMPLE STRUCTURE
RELATIVE FLEXION = 1

SANDWICH STRUCTURE
DOUBLED THICKNESS
RELATIVE FLEXION = 0,140

SANDWICH STRUCTURE
QUADRUPLE THICKNESS
RELATIVE FLEXION = 0,027

Fig. 2 The moment of inertia of a material depends on the cube of the materials thickness

to be able to construct different shapes. Composite materials offer unde-niable advantages over traditional materials from all viewpoints. Fibres can be shaped in any way to produce an infinity of shapes. Making slight adjustments, it is possible to reinforce single parts without weighing down the global structure. The thickness and type of resin used can be optimised for a great variety of needs. The fibres themselves can be oriented in such a way as to follow the main lines of force. Some materials are sold with fibres already in a state of maximum extension, thus producing less stretch and favouring rigidity. There are long and continuous fibres, fibres with the classic single-direction weaving of the weft and warp (fibres follow a geometric pattern but do not interlace), biaxial and triaxial fibres, materials whose short single fibres are arranged in an extended order (called Mat).

Finally, it should be remembered that the moment of inertia of a material, or in very simple terms its resistance to bending stress, grows according to the cube of the material's thickness (Fig. 2). Great thicknesses can of course be obtained using traditional materials, but the price to be paid for such resistance is excess weight. Construction techniques for composite materials make it possible to build "sandwich" structures obtained by sticking two thin sheets, called skins, onto a very thick but lightweight material, called the core (Fig. 3).

The resistance functions of a composite material are chiefly assigned to the fibres, while the resin acts to bind together the various layers of fibre, with the consequent even distribution of stress over the entire structure and its impermeabilisation. It is therefore important to have an adequate resin-fibre ratio in the laminated structure. Excessive use of the former will only produce a rise in weight and a drop in the mechanical properties of the fibre layers. A low amount of resin, or its imperfect distribution, could give delami-

SANDWICH STRUCTURE COMPOSITION

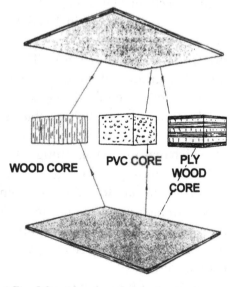

WOOD CORE   PVC CORE   PLY WOOD CORE

Fig. 3 Samples of sandwich structure composition

nation. A great thing that puts composite materials way out in front of other materials is the possibility of orienting fibres in relation to the stress exerted at particular points. Stratification may consist solely of fibres and resin. In this case, we can talk of simple rolled sections. Or it may include an internal layer of another material, thus creating sandwich panels. Both types may then be treated with techniques that magnify its resistance properties, namely vacuum and post-treatment techniques (see below).

Below are brief descriptions of materials and technologies used.

Fibres

There are three sorts of fibreglass: types E, R and S. These have very different resistance properties and production costs. Fibreglass may be produced in Mat form, a sort of "felt" where the short single fibres are arranged in an extended order. The Mat serves as a thickening layer between materials or laths, especially when it is not used, with its particular structure and the considerable absorption of resin, to fill the micro-undulations present on the surface of each layer, and to improve adhesion. Its short fibres do not however guarantee a high degree of resistance. A laminated structure consisting of Mat only will have very similar mechanical properties to those of resin used on its own.

Kevlar 49, discovered in 1965 by Du Pont and available in various material configurations, possesses a high degree of resistance to tensile stress, united with a low density. This means a two-fold saving on weight, since the lightness of the material itself is supplemented by the need for fewer layers required to ensure robustness, which is in any case much greater than that obtainable using fibreglass E. Kevlar is actually five times more resistant than steel, and stretches less than half of steel, for which reason it is beginning to be used for rigging too.

Now commonplace and greatly appreciated among the manufacturers of materials for sails and roping, the "yellow" fibre has proved to be extremely useful in hull lamination activities, increasing threefold the resistance to impacts as compared with fibreglass. The disadvantages of using this material are chiefly the complexity and high cost of its manufacture.

Carbon is a fibre widely used in other sectors, especially in aeronautics and motor racing. Its use in the nautical sector has so far been limited to the competitive sphere. Manufacturers of mass-produced craft still look on carbon with some circumspection due to its high cost (10 times that of fibreglass E) and its low resistance to impacts. Furthermore, if it is to be used profitably, it requires more sophisticated and accordingly more expensive manufacturing techniques. The particular qualities of this material are its tensile strength and pliability, which combine to produce unrivalled rigidity, of fundamental importance for a sailboat. Using carbon to reinforce the hull, it is possible lighten the entire structure by around 40%.

Finally, there are several types of hybrid materials, in which the various fibrous materials interlace to take advantage of the positive qualities of each element. Fibreglass-kevlar and kevlar-carbon are currently the most common of these combinations. The properties of FiberGlass E, FiberGlass S, Kevlar and Carbon Fiber are shown in Fig. 4.

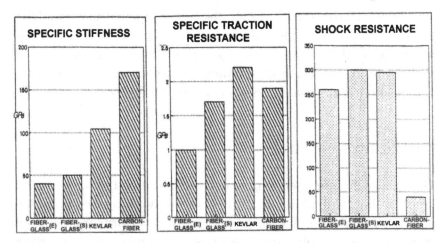

Fig. 4 Specific stiffness, traction, and shock resistance of FiberGlass E, FiberGlass S, Kevlar, and CarbonFiber

Resins

As mentioned above, resistance qualities are chiefly possessed by the fibres of a composite material. Yet the bonding agent too – the resin – must conform to some essential requirements if the entire laminated structure is to be robust. The elongation, or stretch parameter, is of particular importance, needing to be as high as possible. Resin must, without fracturing, act as a "buffer" against the various stresses to which a laminated structure is subjected, working in conjunction with the fibres. The other necessary element is a good bonding capacity to enable the layers of fibre to be perfectly bound together and distribute loads evenly over the entire structure. An imperfect adhesion may lead to the phenomenon of delamination. This is why some less adhesive materials require tougher resins and more sophisticated manufacturing techniques.

Polyester resin is the most commonly used resin in mass production owing to its low cost and ease of use. Compared with vinyl and epoxy resins, the polyester resin has the lowest stretch parameter of the three resin systems. Its adhesion capacity and capacity not to absorb water are also lower.

Finally, although epoxy resin is little used for the mass production of sailboats, it is the resin that offers the best adhesion capacity and the highest stretch ratio, up to four times that of a polyester resin. This is why it is so good at impermeabilising the laminated structure. The use of epoxy resin is also subject to rather laborious post-treatment techniques, and its principal drawback is again its high cost.

Manufacturing methods

The basic technique used to manufacture reinforced plastic is that of simple rolling, with alternate layers of variously configured fibres impregnated with resin. Simple rolling is easy to perform and does not require special or sophisticated techniques. It is relatively inexpensive yet guarantees a good quality for the finished product. The principal drawback is the considerable weight. Lacking in structural rigidity, this material needs to be reinforced by a dense frame of plates and panels.

The sandwich solution is another widely used technique, and has recently revolutionised the way hulls are built. This consists of two relatively thin simple rolled sections, called skins, separated by a thick, lightweight material, called the core. Its main property is its excellent resistance to bending, and is thus able to make a big difference to the structure's rigidity which, as we saw previously, is calculated by the cube of the thickness.

In a rolled section, therefore, the resistance to bending is entrusted exclusively to the properties of the reinforcing agent and properties of the resin. In a sandwich structure, the resistance to bending is increased not only by the properties of the materials used but also by the thickness deriving from the presence of a core. Given the same level of robustness, it is thus possible to make a weight saving of up to 40%, also reducing reinforcements, since the sandwich structure acts as the load-bearing structure. Fatigue resistance also increase thanks to the high capacity to absorb vibrations. Heat insulation is also enhanced using this technique, making the boat less susceptible to temperature fluctuations.

In the points of greatest stress, such as the bulbous bow or the keelson, the two skins meet in simple rolled sections, without the core.

The core may be made from balsa (common balsa or that used in aviation construction), closed-cell PVC ("Termanto", "Cadorite", "Divinycell", "Airex") or honeycomb material (aluminium or aramid fibre, known as "Nomex").

The fundamental requirement of a sandwich structure is the perfect adhesion between the skins and the core, so that the panel acts as a single body. Poor assembly is its weak spot: to avoid this, it is preferable to use a vinyl or epoxy resin and adopt the vacuum technique.

Construction technologies

The vacuum technique, used for many years to construct raceboats, is now being used in mass production in the nautical sphere. It is suitable for sandwich lamination, in that it optimises adhesion between the skins and the core, evenly distributing the bonding agent and infiltrating in the gaps left by the balsa or PVC. But even in a simple rolled section, the vacuum technique has the considerable advantage of removing the bubbles that form between the various layers and of better compacting fibres. It also renders the laminated structure lighter, eliminating excess resin.

Lastly, the post-treatment technique entails the heating of the rolled section at a temperature of 70-100°C for 5/6 hours during the polymerisation phase. This brings about a significant improvement in the mechanical properties of the resin.

The advantages deriving from the use of these elements in terms of rigidity and lightness have thus influenced craft design, and have enormously improved performances, since each of the described properties and the various construction technologies employed have given designers the freedom to experiment as never before in the boatbuilding sphere.

On the other hand, the use of new materials and technologies has brought with it some disadvantages, such as higher costs and, above all, the need to start from scratch, and with great precision, when studying the structural stress to which hulls and boat equipment are subjected.

Some clamorous fractures seen in sailing incidents in recent years must indeed be attributed to mistakes in structural calculations. A prime example was the sinking of the Australian boat during the last America's Cup, but there have also been a number of incidents during ocean-going races that have sometimes brought about the loss of human lives.

Nevertheless, the continuous evolution of sailing and the opportunities offered by new materials, new design and construction techniques and simulation software are the factors that are continuing to add new variables to the problem.

And this helps keep up our interest in studying an art as old as sailing.

References

1. Abbot I.H., von Doenhoff. Theory of wing section. Dover pb., New York 1959.
2. Barkla H.M. The behaviour of the sailing yacht. In abstract of the Royal Institution of Naval Architects, no. 103, 1961.
3. Garret Ross. The symmetry of sailing. Adlard Coles Ltd, London 1987.
4. Kay H.F. The science of yachts, wind and water. Foulis and Co., Henley on Thames, 1980.
5. Marchaj C.A. Sailing theory and practice. Dodd, Mead, and Company inc., New York 1982.
6. Marchaj C.A. Aero-hydrodynamics of sailing. Granada Publishing, London, 1979.
7. Smith Lawrie. Tuning yachts & small keelboats. Fernhurst Books, Brighton, 1988.
8. Wood, C.J., Tan S.H. Toward an optimum yacht sail. Journal of Fluid Mechanics, no. 85, 1978.

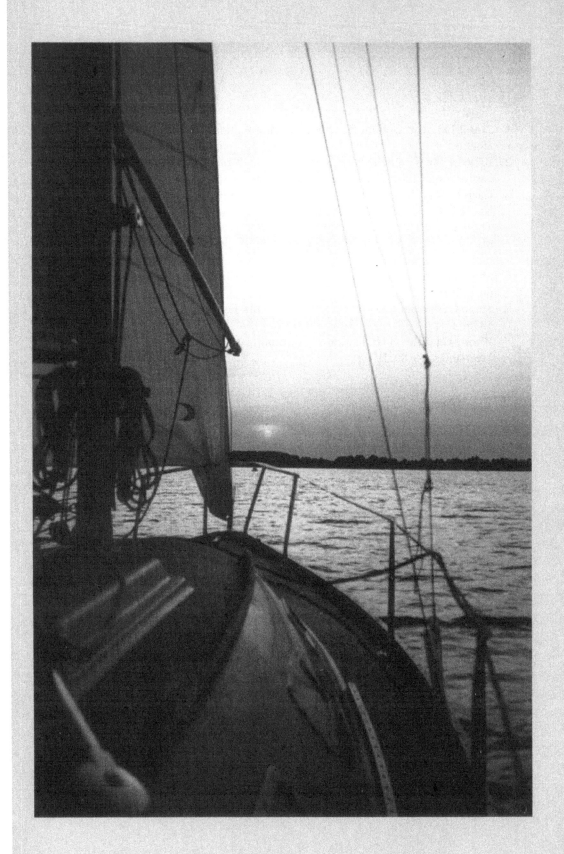

Socio-economic factors in the development of sailing sport technology

Klaus Heinemann

Synopsis

The main theses of this article are, that technology is not only an artifact, but a social institution. It is produced under specific cultural, social, organizational, political etc. circumstances and is has consequences on social behavior and social relations. Following these theses, on the one hand we analyze the origins and development of sailing technology, on the other hand the social consequences, especially as far as the chances in the culture of sailing are concerned.

Introduction

In his book "Sachdominanz in Sozialstrukturen"(The dominance of objects in social structures) (5) Linde highlighted the following important fact, which also applies to the sociology of sport: "objects", as a collective term used to describe the circumstances in which material finds itself and technical artefacts, are man-made; but due to this they become a social institution and a medium of socialisation. They determine behavioural patterns, justify social relations, circumscribe the leeway available in making arrangements, lay down the possibilities for future developments and their shape, and dominate social structures. As a result they have come to have the same importance as social norms like the law, money, and power. The recognition of this fact can be traced back to Durkheim, who Linde refers to. This basic fact, however, has been somewhat forgotten by sociologists.

This "obviousness to objects" (5) is also true for the sociology of sport. This is easy to explain: sporting facilities, apparatus, equipment, and materials were largely standardised in traditional competitive sport, in order to ensure that everyone had the same chance and that the results were comparable. The development of new technology helped (almost) exclusively towards improving sporting performance and registering differences in performance more precisely. In addition, the new technology was characterised by its simplicity, clarity, and the precise definition of its function within the framework of the existing rules. The result of the simplicity was that the sportsman usually possessed the necessary know-how, ability, equipment, and material in order to look after and, if need be, repair their sporting equipment and facilities themselves. The sportsman and the improvement of his sporting abilities and physical and technical competence were the focus of interest, not so much the continual improvement of the technology used in sporting objects.

This situation has changed fundamentally: Sporting activities are increasingly dependent on high-tech products. Their development, production, use, and maintenance require more and more highly specialised technical know-how, professional skills and capital which can no longer be supplied by do-it-yourself or self help organisations. The earlier belief that the type of equipment used was created and promoted within the framework of an established system of rules which varied from sport to sport, and where apparatus, facilities, equipment, clothing, and additional products (such as cleaning products and special foods) were simply derivatives has vanished. Instead the development of these structures in relation to objects has become the independent motor behind sporting development – in accordance with the dominance of objects in social structures discussed by Linde. New technological innovations drive forward the dynamics of development and changes in sport. The way in which sport presents itself and the methods of doing sport are increasingly defined by the provision, acquisition, and use of ever more complex, technologically more advanced and more perfect technical components (apparatus, equipment, facilities, clothing, infrastructure etc.). This technical development has become an independent driving force in the development of sport. I am not talking here about high level sport but about leisure and popular sport.

Technological developments follow their own laws. This can be well demonstrated by a typical characteristic of the sailing technology. What I want to show therefor in this article is, that 1. the technological development is not an automatic process, following an internal logic of technique and engineering but that it is embedded in to a socio-economic and cultural frame which we have to take into account and 2. that the technological development of sailing sport has a tremendous influence on sailing and the specific culture of sailing.

Sport technology and the technologizing of sailing

Before a model of the development of technology in sailing sport can be introduced, it must be clear as to what is meant by "sport technology". The term "sport technology" should constitute the following facts:

1. Sport technology as *"physical objects, or rather technological artifacts to solve problems, that is to say for coping with concrete tasks"* that find their use in the context of sport. However this specification is too rough for our purposes. We must rather differentiate between the following forms of technology:

a. Artifacts used directly while practicing a sport, such as sports equipment, sportswear, special food, sports grounds. One can describe these as "user technologies in sport". Some of these user technologies are integral parts of the practice of sport itself, while others are of service during the preparation before and the evaluation afterwards – such as training equipment, measuring- and viewing devices and medical equipment, including medicine. Still others serve to determine or investigate performance and success. They are thus "instrumental technologies in sport";

b. Artifacts serving as raw- or basis materials for the construction of the objects listed under a. – such as new fabrics, chemical and metal compounds (e.g. GKF, carbon fiber, titanium and the like), new developments in electronics, and in motor technology. These should be called "preparatory technologies";

c. Technological improvements in the processes of production in the manufacture of sport technologies – for instance the processing of titanium and aluminum for equipment, of carbon fibber for masts, of foil for sails and the like. This includes the development of new computer programs for designing yachts, that is to say for the drawing and cutting out of sails. They are thus "process- and production technologies";

d. Scientific discoveries (in terms of natural science and engineering), e.g. in the field of aerodynamics and laws of currents, the courses of combustion in motors, properties of materials, etc.. The results of research on the origin and the fighting of osmosis and on the effects of chemicals that could be used in underwater colors, as well as insights on adhesives can also serve as examples. In these cases one should speak of "basis technologies".

Furthermore we must differentiate within the user technologies:

- single *technological components* – related to sailing ships, e.g. sail, rigging, metal fittings, motors, ropes, anchor, navigational equipment;

- the sport technology like a sailing boat device as a *technological complex* that comes into existence by the fusion of various combinations of different technological components. Such a sports device tends to be developed from a sensible combination of technological elements – the sailing boat out of the boat's body, the motor, the rigging, the sail, navigational instruments, the anchor, winches, metal fittings, etc.. The development of a technological complex "sports device" is a multitude of differently running paths of technological development of each technological component and technological complex, branching off into different directions. Within these, the preliminary decisions for the technological development and form of each respective sports device are made (5).

- the *complex consumer technology*. Every kind of sport is bound to the successful operation of a multitude of technological components and technological complexes that must be linked to one another: sailing, with the technological complex 'sailing boat', marinas, service facilities, sea-maps, the trade with paraphernalia, insurance's, security- systems, learning facilities, weather forecasts, information-systems, etc. Only with this complex consumer technology can the person interested in sport be offered that value of experience and recovery that has made skiing, biking, fitness-sports, sailing, etc. into popular sports (1). The flawless use of sports equipment relies on as perfect as possible a functioning of a complex consumer technology.

Development of technologies as a socio-economic process

If one wishes to trace the social-economic forming of the development of new technologies in sport, one must answer the following questions:
1. Which social, economic, institutional, judicial and organizational factors and interests push the technological development of these thus understood sport technologies?
2. Which new technologies come into existence in this process, or, more precisely, which specific characteristics do they show?
3. Which innovations succeed on the market and are accepted by the user and which innovations prove to be unsuccessful?

The factors taken into consideration to answer these questions are combined in Fig. 1. It thus becomes obvious that new technologies are developed in a socio-economically determined process bound in specific institutional general conditions and in which the various different agents with their differing interests make decisions and interact within technical, normative (partly judicial) and cultural bounds. An institutional economic approach is used to explain the process of technologisation. Thus the thesis will be justified and explained in the following, that every technological development is an open social process formed by (a.) the organizational characteristics of the actors and the institutional arrangements that entangle these, as well as (b.) the technological and cultural givens. A new technology does not come into existence straightforwardly, or determined, or in "one best way", as is associated in Fig. 1. A new technology is the coincidental result of the institutionalized or even informal interaction of different actors in a complex net of influential factors. The development of new technologies is a social project that is realized in this net of different actors influenced by different economical, political and social interests and social givens.

Appropriately the following explanations are structured into three chapters: firstly, the general conditions within which the processes of innovation are carried out (using the example of sailing-technology), introducing the four elements "actors", "institutional arrangements", "technological bases" and "cultural embedding". To build up on that, some characteristics of these processes of innovation are described. Finally, the complex consumer technology "sailing", which is developing under these contexts is outlined with a few brief strokes.

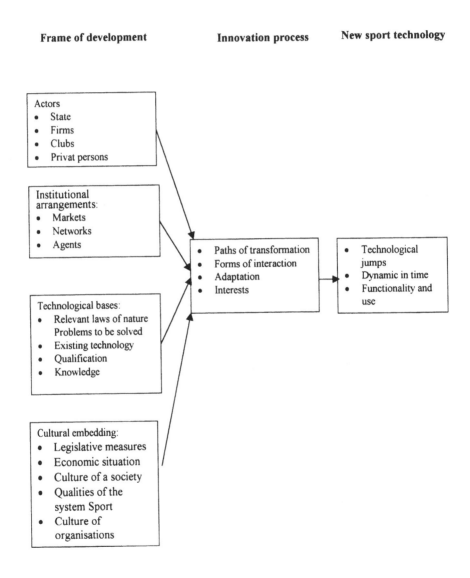

Frame of development   **Innovation process**   **New sport technology**

Actors
- State
- Firms
- Clubs
- Privat persons

Institutional arrangements:
- Markets
- Networks
- Agents

Technological bases:
- Relevant laws of nature
  Problems to be solved
- Existing technology
- Qualification
- Knowledge

Cultural embedding:
- Legislative measures
- Economic situation
- Culture of a society
- Qualities of the system Sport
- Culture of organisations

- Paths of transformation
- Forms of interaction
- Adaptation
- Interests

- Technological jumps
- Dynamic in time
- Functionality and use

Fig. 1 Socio-economic embedding of sport technology development.

General conditions of the process of technologization

General characterization of the general conditions

In the following an attempt is made to answer the above questions and to exemplify in which forms the process of innovation is influenced by the general conditions. Here one can differentiate:

1. The *structural features of the actors,* specific to organizations, differentiating between state, enterprise, unions, users. The following play a role in the dynamics of the process of innovation and the direction it takes:

- The type of <u>decision-making structures</u>: the subject and contents of a decision are fundamentally influenced by the manner in which this decision is made (2). Here one must differentiate between decision-making processes in hierarchical orders (e.g. government or private administration), democratic decisions (thus made by majorities, including in the decision-making process those people who are affected) and individual/family decisions, i.e. the user. Maritime rules, security rules applying to standardization and norm setting (e.g. FM radio broadcasting), work- and environmental security measures (use of non-toxic anti-fouling, installation of fecal tanks), building-regulations to ensure standards of quality and security, establishing formal quality requirements (boating license, broadcasting certificate, license for the use of flare guns) are royally made by the state. This thus often fixes the direction and form of future technological developments. Simultaneously they form the "background of legitimization" of technological artifacts (3). The special thing about this tends to be that such decisions are not specifically aimed at sport matters, especially not sailing, but generally meant for, e.g. the security of shipping, radio communication and the protection of the environment, which sailing must subordinate itself to (often painfully and unwillingly). On the other hand decisions made by unions, that is to say commissions on, e.g., competition rules, measuring regulations, class guidelines and the like – made democratically – are related directly to sailing, that is to say, a specific boat class. The peculiarities of the structures of associations, especially sport clubs/sport federations deserve to have special attention drawn to the characteristic of institutional restrictions of the process of innovation. Firstly, these play a central role as users of sport technologies, often as gatekeepers for the introduction of new sport technologies and the way in which these are used. Secondly, they set rigid handicaps and general conditions for technological development, e.g. with class-rules, by means of building- and measuring regulations for hull, sail, metal fittings and standardization (e.g. of the equipment). Also they establish which materials are allowed and determine contest rules and announced sailing contests.

- The size of the actors' organization: The size does not only help determine each respective development potential, i.e. the economic strength necessary to develop an innovation into a marketable commodity; the technical know-how and the various experiences crucial for the development of high-tech products are more likely to accumulate in larger organizations. Large enterprises also have the opportunity to weave nets with the producers of basis materials, process techniques and the like, to have an influence on their development and to develop and apply new production technologies (as in series production). Finally it is easier for larger organizations, that is to say agents, to impose their creative will on a political level.

- The process of production: For example, shipyards changing to series production are more likely to put through new developments in production, that is to say, they will look for new technologies suited for the production of greater series.

- The organization's culture: For example, the potential of innovation varies, depending on whether the shipyard sees itself as a traditional boatbilder workshop, or as a modern industrial enterprise that happens to earn its money with the building of sailing boats. Furthermore, it depends on whether the decision-makers come from the sailing-sport themselves (mostly regatta sailing) or whether they see themselves as "mere" businessmen and engineers.[1]

- The users: The direction innovation takes depends on whether the users targeted are private (e.g. owners themselves), whether this boat serves as a family- and voyage boat or as a regatta boat, or on the other hand whether the user is a profit-orientated business - i.e. charter enterprises, for example.

2. *Institutional arrangements:* what is meant by institutional arrangements are the forms of agreement and coordination of the various actors active in development, production, sales, care and maintenance of sport technologies. One can differentiate between three different institutional arrangements.

a. Markets, i.e. the coordination of economic actions between suppliers and demanders, by means of free agreements on the price mechanism. The process of innovation can be influenced by:

- the market power of suppliers or demanders. Individual suppliers of high-tech products can have a quasi-monopoly due to their technological competence, as is the case with the manufacturers of winches and masts. But occasionally monopolies can hinder innovation, especially when new developments are costly and risky due to competing suppliers. It is also possible for a monopolist also maintain his existence in a market with technologically obsolete products;

- a multitude of markets, meaning, e.g. the significance of the boat sector, or even merely the sailing-boat sector, for single producers, i.e. also the degree of diversification of the range of products for different markets. For the producers of fiberglass and fabrics the boat sector has become small and insignificant, so that from that side not much pressure can be exerted to show much consideration for its needs;

- the openness of markets; barriers of entry can exist, e.g. when electronic devices for radio-broadcasting, navigation and radar require acceptance by the post in Germany, or when production businesses must fulfill especially strict security requirements, quality standards, health and safety standards, etc.;

- intensity of the competition in and around markets; many suppliers may fight equally over a customer in an existing market, or competition over markets occurs where customers must be won for not yet existing products. New markets require new products to be developed – as was typical of the early '90s, where, with the rapid growth of the charter market, new customers were attracted by new products.[2]

b. Networks, thus defined by the development of long-term relationships between actors. Such networks ensure a stable cooperation, long-lasting access to innovative potentials, knowledge and technological know-how. But in the long run, existing networks may lead to failing to be on a permanent timely lookout for more attractive alternatives.[3]

Networks can:
- be established by means of contracts. This type develops when e.g. a shipyard makes contractual agreements with a constructor who is then responsible for drawing the blueprints for the shipyard over many years. Appropriate connections between producers (shipyards) and their corresponding sales- and dealer organizations are also common.
- grow out of informal or long-run cooperation. Such networks can often be observed between shipyards and individual suppliers (mostly sail-makers and ship motor manufacturers) or charter businesses.

c. <u>Agents</u>. 'Agents' refers to (mostly voluntarily) organized institutions whose purposes are the coordination of the various actors, the standardization of products or processes of production, influencing political decisions, etc.. Especially committees but also umbrella organizations are meant.

3. *Technological bases:* these include:

a. The <u>relevant laws of nature</u>. Aerodynamic laws and natural laws of current- and floating behavior of objects in water are insurmountable frame conditions of technological developments. With innovation one will endeavor to use these laws optimally or even to outwit them. Thus exists a "theoretical hull speed" which, similar to the speed of sound, can theoretically not be passed without a displacer. But with a clever hull construction it is easier to reach this hull speed and under certain circumstances it is easy to pass it. There is great potential for innovation here.

b. <u>Norm settings of tool-technology</u>, as laid down in the corresponding scientific engineering, electro-technical, etc. handbooks and especially in schooling books for boat construction.

c. <u>Qualification</u>. What was primarily important for a long time, was the practical experience of a constructor or a sailmaker. Potentials for development thus used to depend on their collected experience, i.e. the empirically acquired qualification. Further they were limited by the time needed to draw a new hull and to build a boat that fulfilled the future owner's needs. Finally there remained a remarkable risk, because it was hardly ever possible, for cost reasons, to test and optimize in current-canals with a scale model of the design. Thanks to the developments of computer programs for the sail and also the ship's hulls, the situation has fundamentally changed.

d. Knowledge. If one wishes to estimate the influence that knowledge has on the genesis of technology, it is not the total existing knowledge that is of relevance, but that which is actually available to each respective actor.[4]

All respective distribution and availability of knowledge is in turn institutionalized, codified, partly even judicially regulated (patent-rights, education and examination guidelines, job structures) and depends on economic interests. So knowledge must be subdivided according to the following points of view: it can be: a. public, principally available to everyone, or b. private, i.e. available only to one firm or group of people (e.g. professions) or individual people, as firm- or production secrets, empirically gained experience, acquired qualifications, etc. Public knowledge must in turn be divided into knowledge that can be used by everyone and knowledge that is available to everyone but has limitations on its use (e.g. because of patents). If one wishes to use this knowledge, one must pay license fees. But even public and basically freely available knowledge must be adapted and made useable individually. Whoever is in need of knowledge must first find out whether such knowledge exists in the first place, who has what knowledge and how it can be made available. Simultaneously one needs to be able to judge how much this knowledge is worth for the own purposes. The utilization of public knowledge is in turn connected to costs – and whether these costs can be carried in turn depends on the structure of the agents and the institutional arrangements through which one may come by such knowledge.

4. *Cultural and economical embedding.* Agents and their institutional inter-weaving do not exist in a space "devoid of culture". They are rather part of an economy, society and culture and the values, norms and modi of action valid there. These have an effect themselves as economic, cultural and social frame conditions of the technological development. To this we must add:

a. the legislative measures, legal norms (e.g. property protection, pa-tent rights) and conscience of rights (i.e. to have a say in the deve-lopment of special alarm systems for boats, DIN restrictions, VDI and VDE (union of German electro-technicians) guidelines, rules of construction and safety regulations (recently laid down E.C.-wide for sailing boats), stipulations of the North-German Lloyd etc. and tax laws that, for example, open up new write-off possibilities for charter boats bought by private people.

b. <u>Economic situation</u>. The acquisition of a sailing boat is a big investment for most owners, possible only in a favorable economic situation or in a country wherein there exists an appropriate demand due to the acquisitional structure or the inherited fortune. Thus technological developments are sometimes put back, because no spending power can be expected for new products.

c. The <u>culture of a society</u> in which are anchored values like friendliness of technology and experimenting, acceptance of renewals and the insecurity connected to these etc. Here the technology of sport would do well with an orientation (even it were different from country to country), stating that technology and technological progress is useful, helpful, and justified in society. One remains open to new ideas, knowing that what exists at the moment will soon be overtaken by new things.

d. The <u>exceptional qualities of the system 'sport'</u>, or the features of one type of sport, i.e. the specific culture, philosophy and ideology that has developed out of the history and tradition of this type of sport (e.g. sailing). Therefore there exists amongst e.g. sailors a tightly anchored idea of what a "real" sailing boat should look like, and the further development of this piece of sports equipment must orientate itself around this.[5]

These four elements of the frame conditions work together in the process of technologisation. A detailed study depends on deciphering in full how these frame conditions form the process of innovation.

Actors and arrangements in sailing

Fig. 2 illustrates the agents and their interweaving and in how far they are relevant to the development of the complex piece of sports equipment "sailing boat".

With the analysis of this context of coming into existence, the following questions must be answered:
1. Which organizational peculiarities do the different actors have?
2. Which institutional arrangements exist between these actors?

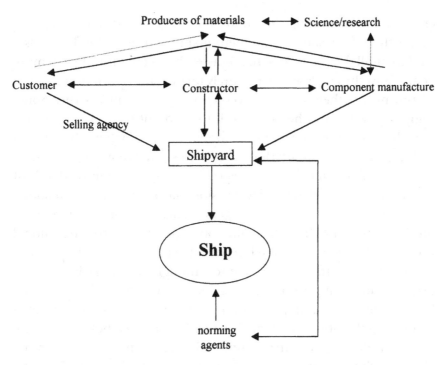

Fig. 2 Context of the coming into existence of the sport technology "sailing".

3. Which interests and motives determine the actors' decisions?
4. Who is in the active, i.e. dominant role in this network of relation-ships?

At this point these four questions cannot be treated referring to all actors. Only the following points are to be mentioned:

The classic equipment producer – e.g. the bicycle factory, the ship-yard, the outfitter of fitness studios – used to be in the position of having the challenge of mostly manufacturing a piece of equipment, including all its components, by himself. But today the single piece of sports equipment has in itself become a complex of highly specialized high-tech products, which the producer can no longer develop further and manufacture on such a high technological level as is demanded. Thus the development, manufacture and maintenance of these components are in turn due to highly specialized firms that have the required tech-nological know-how, the capacities for development and the techno-logies of production. These are often such highly specialized and technologically so extensively developed components, that only very few manufacturers, with a monopolist-like market status construct and supply them. The sports equipment manufacturers – the shipyards – tend to fulfill the purpose of finally assembling the individual components. Most shipyards are increasingly turning into assembly-lines and acquire most of their services and components from third parties. Some shipyards even have the boat's hull formed out of GKF at specialist workshops and the interior installations are manufactured by cabinet-makers, while the shipyards limit themselves to the remaining completion of the ship. However, the degree of branching out or depth of production is in itself a strategic decision that is, up to a point, made by the shipyard's proprietors/managers themselves. On the one hand, there are shipyards (mostly smaller ones, developed from traditional workshops) that target a high level of own production (incl. the ship's construction), with the consequence, though, of not having at their disposal their own potential for the development to the latest techno-logical stand of all components. They tend to survive only in small niches. On the other hand, many shipyards (mostly the larger manu-facturers) develop into the mentioned assembly-lines. But this bran-ching out does not apply generally. Single, larger yacht manufacturers also follow the strategy of greater depth of production, with the conse-quence, though, of quickly isolating themselves economically. Smaller shipyards limit themselves to expert handicraft interior works, using high-quality components obtained elsewhere.

Technologisation of sport as a transformation of technology

In the following, it is to be shown how, within the described framework, new technologies come into existence in a process of transformation. Here transformation does not simply mean, when an idea becomes the starting point for the development of a new product. Transforma-tion is rather a. the process in which new "preparing technologies" or "production technologies" lead to "user technologies"; b. the way in which technological developments outside of sport sinter into sport and c. the way in which new user technologies are assembled to a technological complex: "piece of sports equipment" and integrated

66

into a "complex consumer technology: "sailing", thus completely changing this consumer technology.

In order to understand this process of transformation, 1. the paths on which technological innovations become "user technologies", "technological complexes" and "complex consumer technologies" in sport must be traced; 2. the change that takes place to the new technologies in this process of transformation into a "user technology" must be considered.

Paths of transformation

Paths of transformation refer to the direction taken by a new idea/new product through the various actors, integrated into the existing institutional arrangements, before it becomes a component that is fit for use in the technological complex "sailing boat". Concerning this, one can determine that:

a. The greatest part of innovations in sailing mostly come into existence outside of sailing and even outside of sport. Developments in synthetic materials (like GKF or carbon fibre), developments in the field of electronics – such as GPS, radar –, new fabrics or foils, later used for sails (or sail covers) are developments that have occurred independently of sport and its inferred areas of application. Developments that take place autonomously in sailing are very rare; but even in such cases their further development is dependant on new technologies of production and processing that come into existence outside of sport. Sport is increasingly molded by technological innovations that come from the outside. Provision, acquisition and use of continuously more complex and technologically refined, perfect technological components determine the appearance of sport and the form in which sport is practiced. The technological development has become an independent driving force of the development of sport. This does not only count for top-class sport, but also for leisure- and popular sport. Thus the research of the socio-economic determinants of the development of new sport technologies can also increase our knowledge of the driving forces of the development of sport.[6]

b. The "entrance" for new technologies into sailing is mostly the top-class-, i.e. regatta sport. Reasons for this are that 1. new technologies are mostly adapted to the sport with the aim of increasing the potential performance of regatta yachts and thus increasing their chances of winning, that 2. new technologies are normally very expensive, at least when they are first used, due to high development costs that must be carried by a small number of items. These costs are thus carried by regatta sailors rather than average voyage sailors, for whom the possible gain of performance due to new technologies rather less justifies the high costs, and that. the top-class sport serves as a model insofar as allowing for innovations that have proven themselves in top-class sport, to be commercialized more easily in popular sport. Only few technologies were developed especially, but not exclusively, for popular sports. However one must consider here that by no means all new technologies used in regatta sport will later also find an unbarred entrance to voyage sailing vessels.[7]

Adaptation

Technologies that have developed outside of sport must be adapted to the specific user demands of sailing. This tends to happen in the following ways:

1. *Functional Adaptations:* Technical components must be altered in such a way that the components can withstand the special high pressures of sea that a sailing boat is exposed to – higher danger of corrosion due to aggressive saltwater, high atmospheric humidity, endangering of equipment because of splashwater etc. as well as high and often jerky push- and pull pressures in rough sea and strong heeling over. Moreover the equipment must be (re)constructed in such a way that they also fulfill those (often additional) functions required in sailing – e.g. GPS should not only show the position, but also calculate courses, times and distances to way points and connect these to a map plotter which in turn is combined with other electronic devices (e.g. autopilot).

2. *Differentiation:* Functional qualities are continuously improved and branched out. Every innovation is the starting point of a legion of mutations, with the consequence of a rapidly increasing number of products competing within a class of technical components and sports equipment. Not only is every piece of equipment constantly being improved, but it is also offered with an almost confused multitude of

68

potential performances and possible uses. Thus a differentiation into classes of performance amongst possible uses of pieces of sports equipment becomes visible. – Boats' hulls for regatta ships, voyage- and motor sailing vessels, charterboats – but also for specialized areas of application – rigging for certain areas, metal fittings for the respective user group, equipment and ambience for the corresponding purse etc.

3. *Simplification*: This form of adaptation runs in two directions: one direction is the simplification of operation. Devices are built in such a way that the layman can faultlessly operate them if without great technological knowledge and without effort. Typical for this is the menu-guidance, which takes you through all functions and settings of an electronic device by means of one button. "Sailing on the press of a button" will become an advertising slogan with which a shipyard will offer its highly technologized boats. The second direction is the simplification of maintenance in individual cases. This will be primarily necessary when defects, that is function faults, can occur when no expert repair possibilities are available – i.e. at sea. Winches made by individual manufacturers are a typical example. They are constructed in such a way that they can be disassembled repaired and reassembled in next to no time a few moves without tools. Similar developments become visible in ships motors. Thus user friendliness and maintenance friendliness that bear in mind the requirements and demands of sailing are the directions taken by adaptation.

4. *Miniaturization:* Single components must be built in such a compact and space-saving way that allows for them to be built into and used in the often very tight space also in smaller sailing boats. In addition there is the aim for saving weight, as all additional weight has a negative effect on the potential speed (amongst other things). A typical example is the development of radar, i.e. the radar screen as well as the radar antenna, which must be mounted as high on the mast as possible, with as small a diameter and weight as possible. Thus radar has become an increasingly useable navigational device even for smaller boats. Similar developments can be seen in ships motors: increasingly high performance motors are becoming increasingly compact (and quieter), to also find space in small boats.

Signatures of sport technologies

The sport technologies that develop in this process (again related and restricted to sailing technologies) can be marked by the following, partly contradictory features:

1. *Technological jumps*: by no means do new technologies when they enter the market, i.e. when they are announced as being new, symbolize innovative jumps and fundamental novelties compared to the already existing technologies. The technological development rather takes place in relative small steps rather than fundamental leaps, which leads to qualitatively new technologies. Technological development is an evolutionary process that continuously leads to smaller, step by step improvements, mostly only in the detail. Often they are insignificant changes of already known technologies. Improvements on the potential performance and use are small, if visible at all. In sailing only very few such technological jumps can be noticed to have taken place in the past decades – and here too, one must note that they were no quick, radical changes; new technologies could rather only put themselves through due to long-term resistance.[8]. How is this state of affairs of a step-by-step, evolutional improvement of existing, reliable technologies explained?

Firstly, the conservative position taken by the consumer needs to be mentioned. This should not only be understood in the way that a sailor has firm, tradition-conscious views on what a "good" sailing boat should look like and how it must be equipped; to the average sailor a sailing boat rather symbolizes an enormous investment that one often wishes to use over decades. This dampens willingness to experiment and increases the tendency to fall back on the tried and tested. Specialist trade and the repair trade connected with it often form a further "innovation-brake". They tend only to take over and sell those technologies which they understand themselves, whose uses persuade them and, that they are used to; thus the acquisition of whom they knowingly partake in and for whose maintenance they can also guarantee.

This in turn is at least partially covered with the situation most shipyards are in. Many of those concerned are smaller or medium-sized business. The costs for the development of a new boat are very high. If customers don't accept the innovation, and it thus becomes a flop, this can bring with it massive losses for the shipyard and under certain circumstances even become a threat to their existence.[9] In addition, many businesses have developed out of smaller workshops. These do not always have specialist competence and experience available to them in order to develop or take over innovations themselves. Thus the willingness to experiment is also small.

However, this does not mean that there are only few far-reaching technological innovations to be established within the "consumption technological sailing". These are found less in the user technology and rather more strongly a) in the basis technology, thus in the insights into the behavioral patterns of current, which led to an optimization (and thus optical and technological alignment[10] of boat hulls and sails; b) in the process and production technologies, foremost in the development of computer programs for boat construction etc., in the processing of materials and the series production and c) in the unfolding and optimal combination of the entire consumer technology with all the elements of subject and social systems. Technological developments are thus continuously linked up with organizational and social innovations. The basic and fundamental changes here lie mostly in this branching out and network-like interweavings of a branch of the industry: "sailing".

2. *Functionality and use.* Let us finish by asking what the consumer technology "sailing" that develops under these conditions looks like. To sum up, the following features can be named:

a. Comfort and sportiness: It is said that sailing is sport and that sport has something to do with speed. Thus many shipyards can only exist on the market if their boats have a high potential for speed due to their hull shape, the sail, etc., and can thus be sporty sailed which in this case means fast and high on the wind. But the greater part of owners, because of the following reasons, are 1. seldom in the position and 2. also not prepared to exhaust this potential. Sportiness becomes an image that should be integrated into a shell that is as comfortable and as easy to operate as possible ("sailing on the push of a button") – so that many sporty sailing boats mutate into "floating summer houses" and are used correspondingly: for drinking coffee on the weekends and for a small stroke out of the harbor – as long as the sun is shining and the windforce does not reach over 3 or 4 Beaufort.

b. Simplicity in sophisticated technology: It has already be pointed out that the largest part of technological innovations are aimed at lowering the requests of qualification and competence as well as the physical strain of the user. New technologies enable a "deprofessionalization" of sport. What used to be demanding and often error-prone navigation is now being reduced to the switching on of a navigational computer; the task of reading and interpreting maps has been transferred to a plotter that can also be connected to the autopilot system; the physically demanding operation of the sails has been left to hydraulic winches. Tribulations and hardships of sport are decreasing due to the expansion of the potential performances of new technologies. The direct clash with unfavorable weather conditions is limited by special clothing. New technologies change the meaning and experience of sport. New technologies do not hinder the dealings with risks, the coping with problems of failure and the experience of physical boundaries of performance; however they do make it possible to practice the sport to exclude such possible experiences. The pleasure gained from the perfectly coping with sporty challenges is shifted to the enthusiasm for a clever technology.

c. <u>Risk minimizing with increased risk preparedness</u>: New technologies – navigation, radar, safety technologies of security etc. have the effect that sport can be practiced with less risk and thus becomes accessible to groups of people with less experience, competence and knowledge. Sailing is deproblemized. Two tendencies develop out of this: the willingness for risk rises – on the one hand due to ignorance as to what situations one can get into while sailing, and most of all how to get out of them – further due to the appeal of thrill and adventure – so that despite the technological possible risk reduction, the risk, measured by the frequency of accidents, is not reduced.[11] In addition, the dependence on a reliably functioning technology is increasing. The number of those who rely on complicated technology constantly working faultlessly is increasing; one no longer masters the boat, the navigation, the sail-control. without the use of these technologies. The moment that, e.g. a battery fails all electric devices break down and the clueless skipper can no longer traditionally determine where he is and where he should sail to in order to get into the safety of the harbor. The basic pattern of every such technological development, of increasingly de-problematizing actions by offering perfect solutions to problems – e.g. of navigation – without one having to know how the device works, can become a precarious problem if the device fails and one no longer masters "stone age technology" – e.g. navigation with a sextant.

d. <u>Technological complexity and dependence</u>: High-tech-products had to 1. goods and services that in the past could always be produced 'home-made' can now only be bought. The development manufacture use maintenance and repair of sport technologies increasingly demand highly specialized technological know-how, professional competence and capital that are no longer available as home-made and in self-help organisations. 2. if one produces these goods oneself, one must accept clear losses in the quality of services; the market is offering more perfect and technological complete solutions, which cannot be produced home-made. 3. that home-made manufacture is also becoming increasingly expensive, as it requires more and more expensive technological equipment the use of which also requires high professionality. The practice of sport is increasingly bound to expenses. Home manufacture too demands a constantly growing professional competence and ever increasing investments. Home manufacture is also becoming increasingly capital intensive and professionalised and thus more expensive and, faced with the comparatively low use-intensity and -duration, and less profitable. The sport consumer is becoming increasingly dependent on own specialist competence, or rather competent advice on products which in turn explains the mass of specialist journals related to sport topics, with corresponding product information and tests. It increases the dependence that the layman has on the professional expert.

References

1. Bökemann, D. Bewegungsraum und Sporttourismus – Zur Herstellung und Vermarktung von Sportmilieus am Beispiel des Skilaufs. In: Dietrich, K. & Heinemann, K. (Hrsg.): Der nicht-sportliche Sport.Hofmann Verlag, Schorndorf pp. 211-224 1989.
2. Heinemann, K. Einführung in die Ökonomie des Sports. Hofmann Verlag, Schorndorf 1995.
3. Hennen, L. Technisierung des Alltags. Westdeutscher Verlag, Opladen 1992.
4. Linde, H. Sachdominanz in Sozialstrukturen. Mohr Verlag, Tübingen 1972.
5. Rammert, W. (1994): Techniksoziologie. In: Kerberka, H. / Schmieder, A. (Hrsg.): Spezielle Soziologien,Rowolt Verlag, Reinbek pp. 75-98, 1994.
6. Weingart, P. Differenzierung der Technik oder Entdifferenzierung der Kultur, in: Joerges, B. (Hrsg.): Technik im Alltag, Suhrkamp Verlag, Frankfurt a.M., 145-164, 1988.

Notes

[1] Here one can determine country-specific differences: "Swedish", or rather "Finnish sailing" boat symbolizes a different boat tradition and thus other types of boats than "French" or "English" sailing boat – differences hardly explainable merely because of the different sailing territories that they are primarily built for. By taking this further, one can clarify that the development of the "sailing boat" technology results from these country-specific traditions and the (e.g. skilled trade) qualifications grown out of these, as well as the way boat constructors see themselves; i.e. it is embedded in the respective social environment of the actors.

[2] The building of ships specially for the charter market led to boats a. becoming particularly robust and b. having to offer plenty of space for bunks. This pushed the construction of fiberglass-enforced boat hulls as well as continuously smaller ship's motors and gears.

[3] As an example, I am giving the long-term contractual relationship between a shipyard and a constructor who designed floating caravans rather than 'sport sailing vessels'. This relationship brought the shipyard to the edge of its economical existence

[4] In this context "knowledge" is accepted as being passively present. It must not be overlooked here though, that the further development of technology is in itself "an activity of knowledge production" (6).

[5] Boats tent to heel over with stronger wind, with the desired effect of decreasing the pressure on the sails. But this is in no way ideal, since firstly, the rigging must be set especially firmly, as the entire hull must be pushed to the side with it. Secondly, sailing with strong heeling over is by no means comfortable. Thus more or less brilliant constructions are continuously being produced, with the purpose of only allowing the mast to bend when there is strong wind, while the boat continues to sail in an upright position. but such constructions have never put themselves through on the market, because every sailor "knows" that a boat sailing vertically with a bent mast looks plain ridiculous.

[6] For a long time the many (negative) influences and dangers of an increasingly commercialized sport have been brought to attention in the (mostly sport political and culture critical) discussion. However, it was overlooked that the influences coming from the outside, because of the here mentioned technology of sport, (as) (it is) are at least as great and thus equally remarkable, even if they are guided by economic interests.

[7] As an example I give the sails made out of foil.

[8] 8 deep-reaching changes through the ship-electronics, GPS above all, electronic map-plotters and radar.

[9] As an example for this there is a shipyard known for continuously offering new technological advances in single components in their boats. Hence it was very innovative, but many of these innovations did not reach the expected levels of willingness to buy on behalf of the customer. The firm ended up going bankrupt.

[10] As the boats in the middle class (between 32 and 35 feet) tend to be aligned to one another in the construction and the basis equipment, and also optically due to such technological innovations, this has the consequence of the competition over the customer takes place in the price-arrangements.

[11] Similar tendencies can be observed in skiing, where despite safe technologies (boots, bindings) the number of accidents rises, because – trusting technology – people ski faster and more risky.

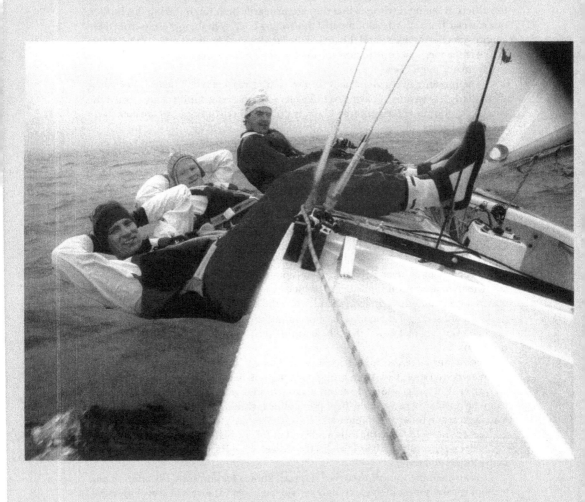

Biomechanics of sailing

Finn Bojsen-Møller & Jens Bojsen-Møller

Synopsis

To maximise the uprighting moment of a dinghy or a small sailing craft the sailors adopt a position called hiking. The effect on the boat of three hiking postures and the biomechanical load on the sailors are described. The demands for strength, endurance and coordination are analysed and recommendations for training activities for seven disciplines of sailing are given.

Introduction

Biomechanics is Newtonian physics applied to living organisms together with the action of living organisms on mechanical events. In sailing the former which might rather be called mechano-biology is the effect of weather, water, and boat on the crew members and their reactions as living persons, while the latter, the proper bio-mechanics, is the physical action of the crew when controlling the boat and the course of the race.

Sailing sets high demands on physical strength, endurance, and agility. As a sport it is unique in combining high level physical activities with a whole body of knowledge of aero- and hydrodynamics, of navigation and meteorology, of general and local sailing conditions including currents and tides, of racing rules and tactics, as well as of the application of hi-tech materials in the standing and running rigging and in the boat.

Sailing also calls for the ability to cooperate, to anticipate events, and to make fast decisions. And finally it takes sensitivity to critical conditions such as the performance of the boat in the water and changes in direction and strength of the wind which can be very subtle and yet decisive.

Though the general conditions: wind, water, boat, crew, and opponents are the same for all classes of boat racing, the actual biomechanical and physiological demands differ quite dramatically from sailboards over dinghies and keelboats to big off-shore boats. Consequently, physical training and personal equipment also differ from class to class. In the following paragraphs we will therefore go through the conditions common to all sailors and subsequently the conditions peculiar to five groups of sailors: dinghy sailors with their hiking position, trapeze hangers, keelboat freeboard hangers (crew), sidedeck hangers (mostly keelboat helmsmen), match racers, and board sailors.

General conditions

An unrestricted moving body enjoys a maximum af six degrees of freedom: three angular movements and three translations. Mathematically, any movement the body performs can be described as a combination of these. While support and stability on land are obtained at the expense of one or more degrees of freedom, a boat at sea will show components of all six. This has been well known among seafarers for a long time and the common nautical terminology actually has names for all six: The angular movements are called rolling, pitching, and yawing, while the translations are termed heaving, swaying, and surging (11) (Fig. 1+2). Fast sailing demands allowance for some of these while others must be controlled. Quite another problem is that the organ of

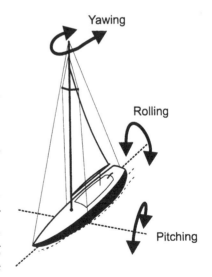

Fig. 1 Drawing of sailboat with three angular movements indicated

balance located in the inner ear of the conventionally land dwelling human being is used to cope with no more than three degrees of freedom at a time. When we set out to sea we are suddenly exposed to six, in some cases with the sad consequence that we develop seasickness.

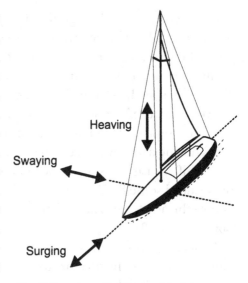

Fig. 2 *Drawing of sailboat with three translatory movements indicated*

Intense exposure to all kinds of weather, rough and cold, calm and burning with ultra-violet light endangering eyes and skin, are among the common conditions that all sailors must deal with. Life jackets, proper clothing, and personal protection against these hazards are indispensable. It is probably less commonly known that the internal temperature of the four big peripheral joints: knee and ankle, elbow and wrist are normally adjusted to about 30-31°C. They tolerate lower temperatures very well but as the joints are cooled down they become stiffer and slower. This is to some degree counteracted by an energy-expensive irrigation of a network of arteries inserted between the joints and the skin. When cold weather is ahead, sailors should add extra insulation inside their sailing suits around the joints before setting out, to protect the joints and ensure the precision and speed of movement for the sailors themselves.

Two more factors must be mentioned under the general conditions. Race sailing in open waters can be a quiet and tranquil affair, but it is often tough, and sailors must train themselves to be strong, endurant, robust, and fast. Long static periods all of a sudden shifts to moments of speed and agility in the handling of sails and keeping the balance of the boat e.g. when tacking or jibing with the spinnaker. To achieve these qualities takes a time consuming and longterm effort.

A less conspicuous but equally important condition is that a good sailor must possess great sensitivity to small changes in the direction and strength of the wind, as well as an acute awareness of how the boat and especially the rudder glide through the water. Subtle changes in the wind can be detected with the eyes, but are often initially picked up by the nose, the ears and the hair of the head and beard. Changes in the driving force is felt in the boat and its degree of heeling, while changes in speed, even small ones, can be heard.

Even out at open sea the wind will veer and back some 5° or 10°, often accompanied by changes in wind speed. This can happen several times during a windward leg and by immediately spotting and utilizing these shifts, gusts and squalls the sailing distance of the upwind leg can be reduced some 8 - 10% or more (11). If the changes are picked up before the adversaries have noticed them a decisive advantage can be obtained (Fig. 3).

A succesful tacking also depends on the crew's feeling for a critically dampened roll of the boat from one side to the other while it instanta-neously gains full driving force.

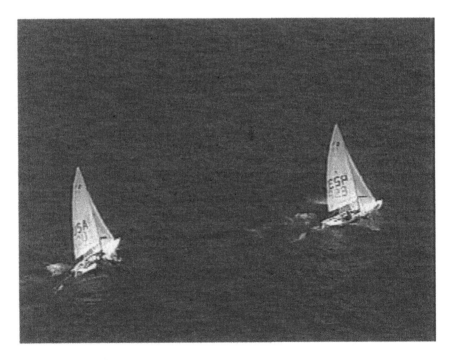

Fig. 3 From the last upwind leg of the Flying Ductman regatta at the Olympic games in Barcelona in 1992. The Spanish boat has captured a slight change in the direction of the wind and is sailing 10-15° higher than its American opponent. After this incident the Spanish boat took a decisive lead and won the gold medal.

Dinghy sailors and the hiking position

In dinghies and small crafts where the weight of the crew relative to that of the boat is large (between 1:1 and 1:4), the position of the crew is important for the balance and uprightness of the boat and thereby for its ability to plane. To maximise the uprighting moment the sailor or sailors adopt a position called the hiking position where they hook their feet under a strap inside the boat and extend their bodies over the sidedeck to windward (7). Hiking is used in close hauled sailing in moderate to high winds.

In the literature and in experiments where the hiking position is transferred to the laboratory it is often characterised as a static position. Accordingly static endurance training is recommended for sailors. However, a small craft moving in the sea is exposed to quite large accelerations up and down and fore-and-aft, whereby the position assumes a dynamic element as well (16, 17).

The crew constitutes a kind of smart balast which shifts the center of gravity of the total system (boat and crew) to preserve the longitudinal as well as the lateral balance. The driving force acting at the sail center and the resisting force from the drag of the wet surface and the keel create a moment that must be balanced by the pair of vectors from the center of buoyancy and the center of gravity (Fig. 4). As a boat heels

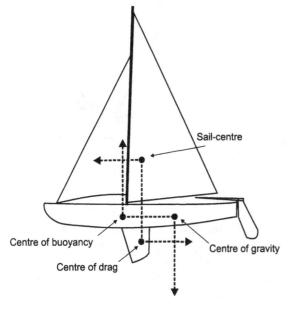

Sail-centre

Centre of buoyancy

Centre of drag

Centre of gravity

Fig. 4 The driving force from the sail center and drag from the center of drag constitutes a pair of vectors giving the boat an anticlockwise pitching moment. They are counteracted by two forces acting at the center of buoyancy and the center of gravity. By moving longitudinally in the cockpit the crew can change the distance between the two latter centers and thus tune the clockwise moment to a perfect balance.

over, the driving force develops a downward directed component which makes the passage of the boat increasingly heavy (Fig. 5). To plane, the dinghy must be kept almost upright. No more than 10-20° heeling is allowed. The righting moment can be increased by hiking whereby the center of gravity moves windwards while the center of buyoancy because of the heeling over at the same time is moved leewards. The force arm is accordingly enlarged in both directions compared to a near neutral upright position (Fig.6 A+B).

In general there are three different hiking or hanging postures (Fig. 7 A, B and C) which can be chosen depending on the available space in the dinghy and the strength and endurance of the sailor. Posture A where the sailor is supported under the thigh is the most frequently used by

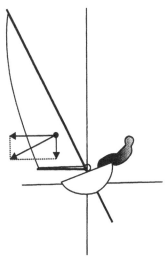

Fig. 5 As the dinghy heels over the driving force develops a downward directed component making the passage through the water increasingly heavy. To plane the dinghy must be kept almost upright by the lateral positioning of the sailor.

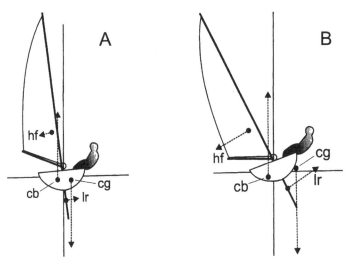

Fig. 6 The driving force and the lateral resistance force are balanced by the forces acting at the center of buoyancy and the center of gravity (A). Increasing wind makes the boat heel over (B). This is counteracted by increasing the distance between the the center of buoyancy which moves leewards as the boat heels, and the center of gravity which moves windward as the crew extends over the sidedeck.

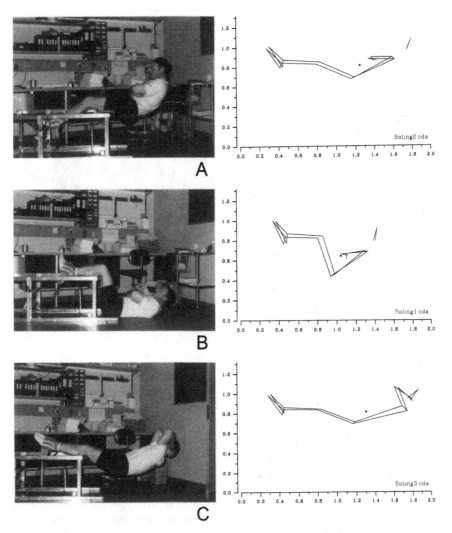

Fig. 7 Three different hiking postures investigated in a test bench and with corresponding stickfigures with the calculated center of gravity shown. The axis of abscissas gives the distance of the center from the centerline. A) shows the sidedeck hiking, B) the freeboard hiking, while C) is the extended sidedeck hiking with the knees stretched and the arms behind the neck.

dinghy sailors and -helmsmen. It is also used by helmsmen in small keelboats. Posture B is used by the crew in Solings and other boats with a freeboard the sailors can "sit" on. Posture C where the knees are extended and the body supported by the knees or upper shank is extremely strenuous and can only be held for a few – maybe 4-5 - minutes. It is called active hanging and is used in especially stressed phases of a race such as the start where everybody is fighting for free wind.

For a group of five Danish male sailors with their arms resting on the chest, a righting moment arm of 1.27 and 1.10 m was found for position A and B respectively (4). The obtained righting moments depend on the height and weight of the sailors, the position of the center of buoyancy in the actual boat, and the actual degree of heeling. Values of 1000-1200 Nm per sailor in the Soling class (Fig. 8) (4) and 800 Nm for a group of Australian elite Laser dinghy sailors (3) have been reported. The effect of the three postures can be increased a further 3-4 % by extending the arms to the level of the head (4) which of course is only possible for crewmen.

The hiking position has been analyzed on test benches in several laboratories in both static positions and under simulated sailing. Putnam (14) found average righting moment arms of 1.16 and 1.08m for positions similar to po-

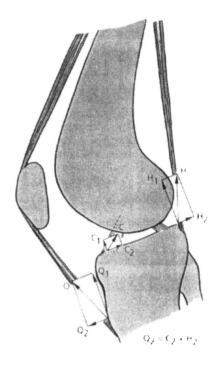

Fig. 8 Drawing of the knee with the effects of the quadriceps (Q) and the hamstring muscles (H) indicated. The quadriceps has an anterior shear component (Q2) which loads the anterior cruciate ligament (C). The hamstring muscles have a posteriorly directed shear component counteracting the anterior shear. A relatively strong co-contraction of the hamstrings seems necessary for relieving the anterior cruciate ligament.

sition A and B. Knee and hip torques are large and can reach 50 % (13) and at the knee even 80-90 % (12, 14) of the maximal voluntary isometric torques. Under static laboratory conditions, knee extension and hip flexion moments of approximately 250 and 200 Nm, respectively, were found depending on the degree of outstretching and the position of the support from the sidedeck (5, 12). Aagaard et al. (1) found a potential of 330 Nm maximal voluntary isokinetic extension moment in the knees in a group of Danish elite sailors. This potential seems easily exploited when hiking at sea.

The reported values all show that the knees are highly loaded in sailors who hike. This applies not only to the joint between the thigh and calf (the femurotibial joint) but also to the joint between the knee cap (the patella) and the thigh (the femur). With a knee flexion of 30° and a moment of 216 Nm in a leg extension exercise, Steinkamp et al. (18) found that the patellofemoral joint reaction force was more than 4.200 N corresponding to a compressive stress of almost 14 MPa over the contact surface. These are very high values but are probably reached time and again in a moving boat with added vertical accelerations. Sustaining such loads for long periods of time together with exposure to cold could easily explain the pain in the knee region, both so-called retropatellar pains and inflammations along the patellar attachment of the infrapatellar ligament, which many sailors complain of (15).

With a knee flexion of 30°-50° the strong quadriceps muscle of the thigh also has a substantial anterior shear component which strains the anterior cruciate ligament inside the knee (Fig. 9). This anterior shear force is counteracted by a co-contraction of the hamstring muscles which thereby offer an important stabilization of the joint, especially in fast knee extensions. To describe this factor Aagaard et al. (1) defined a

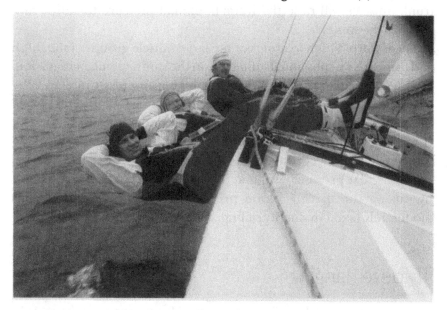

Fig. 9 Hiking in a Soling. The two crewmen sit on the freeboard with their torsos supported by a belt and with their arms behind the neck. The helmsman sits on the sidedeck in a more upright position which brings him within reach of the tiller and gives him a better look-out.

functional hamstring to quadriceps strength ratio, in which "functional" means concentric quadriceps to eccentric hamstring strength, as these two in reality are combined. They found that the elite sailors had a significant potential for muscular knee joint stabilization despite their extremely high quadriceps strengths.

However, as mucles become fatigued their strength, coordination, and cooperation are reduced to unknown degrees with potential emergence of hazards to the structures they should stabilize and protect. This is an important point as a race can take up to three hours and a regatta has two or three races a day plus the time taken to sail out from the habour and back again.

The Laser is a one-man dinghy. Because of the shallow hull the sailor hikes with more extended knees which loads the patellofemoral joint less. In a test bench-simulator which made the sailor perform flexion-extension movements at the hip and knees (range +/-10°) peak moments of 150-200 Nm were obtained (5).

Hiking also involves the trunk muscles. Thus, the lower spine is held by the iliopsoas muscle while the upper part depends on the anterior trunk muscles, especially the rectus abdominis. In action, the trunk muscles will raise the intraabdominal pressure to stiffen and stabilize the spine.

The reported high loadings of the large muscle groups of the thigh and trunk have a substantial influence on the cardiovascular circulation. During simulated as well as on-water hiking the heart rate and the blood pressure were seen to rise steadily and reach high values while the corresponding oxygen uptake only rose moderately (3, 17, 19, 20). It was assumed that the local blood circulation in the large hiking muscles was reduced due to mechanical compression by the high intramuscular pressure, and that the organism tried to overcome this by raising the driving blood pressure. Aerobic capacity is only moderately taxed in dinghy sailing.

Trapeze hanging

In trapeze hanging the sailor is supported from the top of the mast by a belt at the waist while he is standing on top of the freeboard. In this situation he experiences vertical as well as fore-and-aft accelerations in parallel with the boat. Being supported by the trapeze there is no demand for muscle moments at the knees or the hip except to stabilize the posture. Marchetti et al. (12) investigated the biomechanics of trapeze hanging and compared it to hiking. By electromyography notable activity was found only in the sternocleidomastoideus holding the head and neck, the trapezius fixating the shoulder girdle, and the gastrocnemius enabling a tip-toe stand to extend the center of gravity a few last centimeters.

Keelboat freeboard hanging

In keelboats with a vertical freeboard the sailors can adopt a hanging style where they sit on the side of the boat with their torso supported by a belt (Fig. 9). The arms are held behind the neck, which extends the center of gravity a few percent but also relieves the sternocleidomastoideus muscles for holding the head. In the test bench it was found that the resulting righting moment was 13-14% less than at proper hiking (Fig. 8), a value that will depend on the degree of heeling (4). But as the position also is less demanding it is possible to sustain it all the way from the leeward to the windward mark, and for as many races in the regatta as necessary.

Keelboat sidedeck hanging

Sidedeck hanging is a variant of the general hiking position and is usually adopted by the helmsman. The torso is typically more upright with a more kyphotic spine (Fig.9) which strains the passive tissues of the spine but also has some advantages in larger force arms for the muscles around the hip and back. The uprightness allows for a better look-out and a proper distance to the tiller and the mainsheet.

The kyphotic position of the crew and especially of the helmsman exposes the low back, and among smallboat-class sailors Schönle (15) found an increase in the rate of low back pain when the ratio of sail area per crew member increased. A relatively large sail area per sailor increases the need for effective hiking with consequently relatively large loads to the knee, hip and low back. Large sails are heavy to adjust and this hauling aft of the sheets is often done inside the boat in a forward bent position. In simulated dinghy sailing Blackburn (3) found peak mainsheet loads of 5-600 N while in large off-shore boats they can amount to 50-70% maximal voluntary low back extension, probably close to two thousand N (8). The latter loads the lumbar spine equally although differently than when hiking.

Another concern for the helmsman is the necessity to look forward and thus to hold the neck in the same twisted position for long periods. We have found no indications in the literature of an accumulation of neck pain among helmsmen, but troubles in this area seem likely.

Match racers

Match racers adopt all the above described positions. Characteristic for match racers are however the frequency of the sailing manoeuvres. Within the four minutes before start they can tack and jibe 10 to 15 times, in a windward beat of 10 minutes another 10 to 20 tacks can be seen, and in a close race run maybe 10 jibes with the spinnaker in a row. In strong winds the many manoeuvres set high demands on strength, endurance, and agility as well as on the ability to combine strategic anticipations and fast decisions.

Board sailors

Sailboards differ from small dinghies in the mechanical joint which is interposed between the hull and the mast. Because of this there is no uprighting moment from the centers of buyoancy and gravity. Stability is exclusively achieved through balance between the wind pressure and the opposite pull from the sailor. The sailor stands erect, often with the pelvis protruded and with a certain lordosis of the lumbar spine. The exposed muscles are the erector spinae, the superficial back and neck muscles, the stabilizers of the scapula, and the shoulder muscles. In olympic competitions dinghy sailors are only allowed to make three pumping movements with the sail to start planing while the windsurfers have free pumping which they can utilize in light winds very effectively. Pumping is done with a pull-and-push movement in which the anterior shoulder muscles also are engaged. Windsurfing in high winds and with pumping in light winds is an endurance sport with much higher demands on aerobic capacity than is necessary for dinghy sailing, at least in elite sports (5). Exposure to cold, the often long lasting erect posture with a lordotic lumbar spine, together with the heavy load on the back muscles are taken as factors leading to low back complaints among these sailors (10, 16)

Physical training of specific categories of sailors

As previously noted, many factors other than the physical fitness of the crew determine the winner in elite sailing. In some disciplines such as off-shore sailing in large keel-boats, the fitness of the crewmen is of less importance, whereas it is crucial in dinghies and in board-sailing and especially so in high winds.

In all race classes except boardsailing it happens that large 6-day regattas sailed in light and fluky conditions are won by a completely physically unfit sailor. Therefore every sailor must decide how much time to spend on physical training, as the trade-off lies in the fact, that time spent on physical training is time lost for developing gear, tuning the boat, or making other preparations.

In spite of these implications, the mentioned studies and experience suggest that some level of physical fitness is essential. The crucial decision has to be made as to what kind of training would be appropriate to meet the exact needs of each sailing discipline so that no time is "wasted".

The special physical demands for a number of sailing disciplines are suggested below, and can be used to determine which kind of training is recommendable. The suggestions are based on a number of studies on elite sailors of different nationalities (1, 2, 6, 9, 13, Bojsen-Møller unpublished results on Danish and Australian international elite sailors 1998).

A pattern emerges implying that the more the crew to yacht weight ratio decreases, the less the importance of exellent physical fitness. This relationship is primarily due to the fact that the heavier yachts have keels and thus possess a very high stability in themselves. They are not as easily manoeuvered around and balanced off by body weight displacement as the light dinghies are. The forces exerted on the sheets and guys grow large in big yachts hereby to some extent eliminating the possibility of pumping and adjusting the sails rapidly. Heavy yachts do not require hiking nor is it allowed in the racing rules. With heavier

Table 1

Type of sailor:	Sidedeck dinghy hikers	Trapeze sailors	Freeboard hikers	Sidedeck keelboat hikers	Match racers (crew)	Board sailors	Off-shore large keelboat sailors
Type of yacht:	Europe, Finn, 470, Laser	470, 49'er, Tornado crew	Soling & Star crew	Soling & Star helmsmen	Medium to large keelboats	Olympic and other classes	Large to very large keelboats
Max. strength, upper body	good	good	excellent	good	good	good	good
Max.strength: abdomen, lower back,	excellent	good	good	good	good	good	fair
Max.strength:hip flexors, leg's H/Q	excellent	good	good	good	good	good	fair
RFD: explosive strength, fast reactions	good	excellent	good	fair	good	good	fair
Hiking endurance	excellent	-	good	good	-	-	-
Aerobic endurance	good	good	fair	fair	fair	excellent	fair
Coordination	excellent	excellent	good	good	good	excellent	good
Agility	excellent	excellent	good	good	good	excellent	good

Table 1 Physical demands for seven disciplines of sailing. Each fitness parameter is rated in three levels of importance relative to the sailor:

- excellent, meaning that this parameter is of major importance to the sailor and must be as high as possible,
- good, meaning that this parameter must be substantially higher than in normal untrained individuals, but not necessarily near the top figures measured in other elite sports,
- fair, meaning that the sailor is fit enough at normal or above normal levels.

RFD: Rate of force development

Table 2

Goal	Type of training	Training principle/dosis	Side effects
Maximal strength	Strength training, weight machines or free weights	Fairly heavy, highly dependent on former strength training experience and level; 2-5 sets of 4-10 repetitions with 1-2 minutes breaks	Increased body weight, but not necessarily!
RFD: explosive strength, fast reactions	Heavy free weight training, plyometrics	RFD is a quality not traditionally linked to yachting, but maybe important in board sailing and 49'ers	Risk of damaging knees and back. Speak to a professional weight trainer
Hiking endurance	Hiking	Minutes & hours in the hiking strap in the boat, in the "home hiking bench" or training machine	Risks of knee and back pain. Combine hiking training with strength training of hamstrings, lower back and abdominals
Whole body aerobic training	Running, rowing ergometer, aerobics, cycling, circuit training, swimming	Vary between high and low intensity after experience and season. Involve whole body.	Weight loss, but not necessarily
Weight gain	Strength training and eating	Strength training with varying heavy and light weights. Fatiguing the muscles seems to be the building stimulus. Watch out for the ideal weight for the class.	Increased strength
Coordination	Coordination exercises	Jumps, leaps, ball games, gymnastics, aerobics, dancing, sailing a small course without a rudder.	Fun and teambuilding
Agility	Stretching	Stretching on water before and after racing, on land before and after training.	Lower risks of injury?

Table 2 Suggested training to achieve the fitness parameters and levels given in Table

yachts and longer (off-shore) races emphasis lies on tactics and sustained boat speed rather than fast manoeuvres. An important exception is match racing which can be quite physically demanding even in very large yachts.

It is not possible to give specific and detailed training instructions here, but Table 2 offers a selection of training methods designed for achieving the fitness parameters allocated in Table 1 to seven categories of sailors.

As sailing over the last decades has become more professionalised, sailors have been forced to take up physical training as part of their preparation, and as the table shows there are many areas of fitness training, which in the right combination, will give the fit sailor an edge, especially on windy days.

References

1. Aagaard P., E.B.Simonsen, N.Beyer, B.Larsson, P.Magnusson, M.Kjær: Isokinetic Muscle Strength and Capacity for Muscular Knee Joint Stabilization in Elite Sailors. Int. J. Sports Med., 18:521-525, 1997.
2. Aagaard P., N.Beyer, B.Larsson, M.Kjær: Isokinetic Strength and Hiking Performance in Danish Olympic Sailors. Scand. J. Med.Sci.Sports, 8:65-72, 1998.
3. Blackburn M.: Physiological responses to 90 minutes of simulated dinghy sailing. J.Sports Sci., 12:383-390, 1994.
4. Bojsen-Møller J.: Active hanging style (in Danish). Master's thesis, University of Copenhagen, Denmark. P.1-19, 1995.
5. DeVito G., L. Di Filippo, F.Felici, M.Marchetti: Hiking mechanics in laser athletes. Med.Sci.Res., 21:859-860, 1993.
6. De Vito G., L.Di Felippo, A.Rodio, F.Felici, A.Madaffari: Is the Olympic Boardsailor an Endurance Athlete? Int. J. Sports Med., 18:281-284, 1997.
7. Elvstrøm P.: Expert Dinghy Racing. Adlard Coles, London. p. 1-, 1964.
8. Felici F., B.Ricci, G.De Vito, L. Marini, L.Di Felippo, M.Marchetti: Spine loading involvement in off shore sailing. Med.Sci.Res., 21:847-849, 1993.
9. Larsson B., N.Beyer, P.Bay, L.Blønd, P.Aagaard, M.Kjær: Exercise Performance in Elite Male and Female Sailors. Int. J. Sports Med., 17:504-508, 1996.
10. Locke S., G.D.Allen: Etiology of low back pain in elite boardsailors. Med.Sci.Sports and Exercise, 24:964-966, 1992.

11. Marchaj C.A.: Sail Performance, Theory and Practice. Adlard Coles Nautical, London, p. 1-401, 1996.
12. Marchetti M., F.Figura, B.Ricci: Biomechanics of two fundamental sailing postures. J.Sports Med., 20:325-332, 1980.
13. Niinimaa V., G.Wright, R.J.Shephard, L.Clarke: Characteristics of a successful dinghy sailor. J.Sports Med., 17:83-96, 1977.
14. Putnam C.A.: A mathematical model of hiking positions in a sailing dinghy. Med. Sci. Sports, 11:288-292,1979.
15. Schönle C.: Pain and joint stress in sailing. Med. Sci. Res., 21:875-880, 1993.
16. Shephard R.J.: Biology and Medicine of Sailing. Sports Med., 23:350-356, 1997.
17. Spurway N.C., R.Burns: Comparison of dynamic and static fitness-training programmes for dinghy sailors – and some questions concerning the physiology of hiking. Med.Sci.Res., 21:865-867, 1993.
18. Steinkamp L.A., M.F.Dillingham, M.D.Markel, J.A.Hill, K.R.Kaufman: Biomechanical considerations in patellofemoral joint rehabilitation. Am.J.Sports Med., 21:438-444,1993.
19. Vogiatzis I., N.K. Roach, E.A.Trowbridge: Cardiovascular, muscular and blood lactate responses during dinghy 'hiking'. Med.Sci.Res., 21:861-863, 1993.
20. Vogiatzis I., N.C.Spurway, J.Wilson, C.Boreham: Assessment of aerobic and anaerobic demands of dinghy sailing at different wind velocities. J.Sports Med.Phys. Fitness, 35: 103-107, 1995.

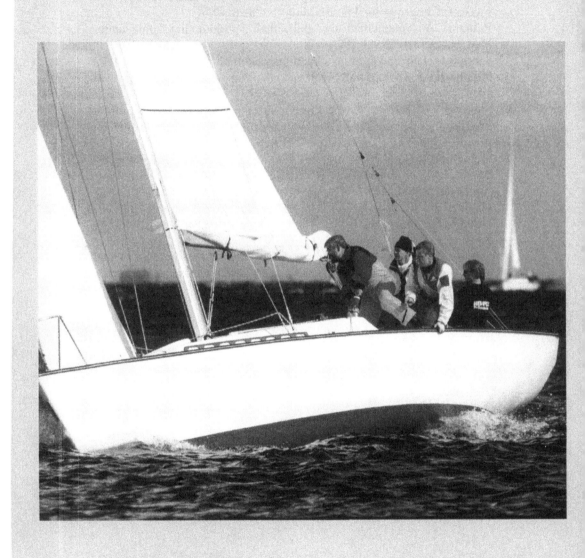

Sailing Physiology

Neil Spurway

Synopsis

Keelboat sailing, boardsailing, dinghy trapezing and dinghy hiking are separately considered. Though matters like breathable fabrics and seasickness are briefly discussed, the emphasis is on the muscular and biomechanical demands of the respective activities, and the nature of the cardiorespiratory challenges resulting. The aims of the sports scientist's contribution must be to minimise the accumulation of chronic stress when sailing, and optimise the efficacy of off-water training. Boardsailing and hiking impose the most continuous physiological demands, but it is argued that they are of importantly different kinds: boardsailing is an essentially dynamic activity, ranking high in the aerobic intensity range, but available evidence indicates that the aerobic requirement of hiking is only half as great, the predominant muscle involvement being 'quasi-isometric'. This contrast should be recognised in training.

Introduction

In this chapter I shall divide sailing into four categories, and treat them in the order:
- i) Keelboating (yacht sailing)
- ii) Boardsailing (windsurfing)
- iii) Dinghy sailing with trapeze
- iv) Dinghy sailing without trapeze.

It is on topic (iv) that I have done most research myself. Further-more, this is the only one upon which there is any degree of contro-versy. For comparative reasons, however, it will be better to discuss the other topics first.

Keelboating (i)

Heeling and Hull Movement

Sailing craft with fixed and heavy keels, whether 6 or 60 metres long, can lie safely at moorings with no-one aboard — which is how the over-whelming majority are normally kept. Because the keel does not begin to exert its righting moment, bringing the hull back towards upright, until displaced from the centre line, in any breeze at all these boats sail somewhat heeled. Nonetheless, crew weight is of at most secondary importance in reducing heel, and nothing more adventurous than sit-ting facing outwards on the windward gunwale is expected of the crews of deep-water racers, or other yachts which are fully decked or cabined. Only in a few small racers with open cockpits, such as Stars and Solings, is sitting out the other way, with one's back over the water ('hiking') necessary. Hiking such keelboats is little different from hiking dinghies (except that it tends to be less comfortable), so I shall defer discussion of it till section (iv).

The postural challenge which confronts all keelboat sailors, as a downside of the fact that their boats cannot be held upright, is the need to move around on a heeling deck or cabin floor. Often this floor will simultaneously be rolling transversely and pitching fore-and-aft, and the gymnastic skills required to crew them effectively are conside-rable. Balance, flexibility and strength are all at a premium. There is surely scope for research into how to acquire these skills most rapidly and completely, and how best to train in advance for the kind of fitness required? Performance and safety, whether on a Whitbread race around the world or a single-handed Atlantic challenge, could both be improved thereby. As yet, however, I know of no such study. Instead, improve-ments have been left to yacht designers, optimising layout; to equipment manufacturers, with their hooks, harnesses and safety lines; and to the pharmaceutical industry, which fortunately continues to see potential profit in the search for improved prophylactics against seasickness.

Meanwhile, non-confidential work on seasickness continues to appear in the literature. Pingree & Pethybridge (26) confirmed many people's subjective impressions by a double-blind sea trial which showed that scopolamine (hyoscine) was more powerful than the antihistamine cinnarizine, not only in protecting against seasickness but in inducing drowsiness and other side effects. More surprising to scientific sceptics will be the finding by Bertolucci & DiDario(3) that the Relief Band (TM), applied at the specified acupuncture point, suppressed symptoms very significantly ($p<0.01$). As to the differences between individuals, making some so much more prone to seasickness than others, there is disagreement whether the vestibulo-ocular reflex has higher gain in susceptible people(15,29), but Gordon et al(15), who find in favour of this postulate, are clear that the frequencies of the simple harmonic motion tests at which the difference shows are crucial: they centre around 0.02—0.04 Hz, in the subjects studied. (One wonders whether, if these subjects had been divided into those most prone to sickness in large vessels and those who suffer worst in yachts, the critical frequencies would have been different for the two groups?) Finally, however, the robust seadog, who has no doubt that seasickness susceptibility correlates with personality, might be surprised by the finding of the same research team (14) that a sample of 25 non-susceptible subjects had significantly *higher* psychoticism scores (assessed by the Eysenck Personality Questionnaire) than the 29 who were very susceptible to *mal de mere*!

Thermoregulation

Another physiological challenge to which the main, practical answers have to be technological rather than biological is that of thermoregulation. Sufficient intakes of fluid in the heat and of calories in the cold are the only biological prescriptions which can effectively be offered. Apart from these, the sailor relies below deck on the designer, to provide good ventilation in hot weather and insulation against cold; modern yachts may be no better insulated than their wood-built predecessors, but those designed for warm latitudes are much better ventilated. Above deck, modern breathable materials have revolutionised the feasibility of keeping the sea out without all one's sweat being kept in. They rely on microporosity in the permselective layer, laminated between abrasion-resistant woven outer and wick-action inner coatings. One of the highest-technology materials has over 10 (9) hydrophilic pores per cm^2. Each pore's diameter is about 25 times greater than that of a single water molecule, yet about 1/150th that of a typical water droplet (data from Henri-Lloyd technical leaflet): thus vapour can pass yet liquid water is fairly effectively excluded. Under such breathable outer garments, the wearer's body heat should be affected by rain and spray only insofar as water cools the clothing's surface.

Many technological developments in the insulating materials themselves have also occurred and are continuing. To see the purpose of one which I find particularly interesting, consider the experience familiar to everyone who has sailed, climbed or skied in cold weather — that the more natural-fibre garments one wears, the less effective each seems to be. A major factor in these diminishing returns is that the inner layers are compressed by the weight of those outside them, squeezing out the air upon which their insulating characteristics depend. The better that cellular materials can be made to resist compression, the fewer, lighter and more flexible the necessary layers will be.

Working at Winches

Many yachtspeople damage their backs. Winchwork and heaving on lines are almost certainly the predominant causes for racing crews. Anchor handling is a major additional threat on cruising boats. In all instances, the loads involved are gravely compounded by the body positions people so often adopt — spines being usually bent forward, and sometimes axially rotated too. Designers could do more to help than they usually do: the 'coffee grinder' winch, of 12 metre and other large yachts, is not only a better biomechanical design, but usually more kindly positioned than the horizontal-action winches which bristle round smaller yachts' cockpits. Anchor-handling gear could undoubtedly be much improved too, if the sailing community had the perception to demand this.

Meantime, it is amazing how much we can help ourselves, where the geometry of the boat allows, by simply pulling with a straight back rather than a bent one. Felici and colleagues (11) modelled torsional moments about the L4/L5 intervertebral joint of a crew member, seated on deck with feet braced against a bar, and showed that the same force

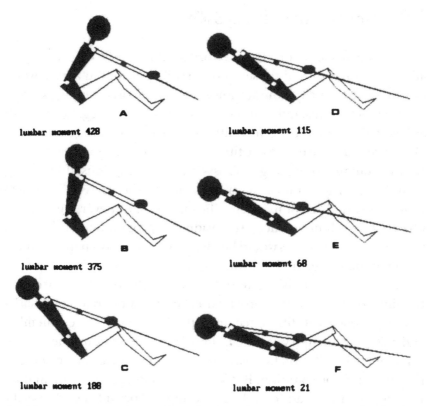

lumbar moment 428

lumbar moment 115

lumbar moment 375

lumbar moment 68

lumbar moment 188

lumbar moment 21

Fig 1 Lumbar moments for seated rope-hauling: the moment in position F is less than 1/20th that in position A. From Felici, F, et al, Spine loading involvements in offshore sailing. Med Sci Res *21, 847-849, 1993. With permission.*

could be exerted on a rope with only 1/20th as great a moment when the back was straight as when it was maximally bent forward (Fig. 1). In the latter case, the moment was similar to those measured in weight lifting exercises: typical weight *training* would impose strains only about 2/3 as great! An apparent paradox was that electromyograms (EMGs) recorded from the erector spinae muscles were less with the most-bent posture than in intermediate trunk positions, but this could be explained if the main load in the fully flexed position was exerted by ligaments, rather than muscles. The distorting forces on the intervertebral discs would be just as severe, whichever their source.

It is appropriate to recognise that, when we have to pull while standing or kneeling, less difference can be made to the lower-back moments than in the position studied by Felici et al. Nevertheless, common sense can still be applied with profit.

Physical Training for Keelboat Sailing

Too few yacht sailors make any effort at all to get fit before they go afloat. But what should those, who are willing to put in a little work, actually do? Specificity is the keynote of modern sports training practice, so we ought to be instantly warned against reliance on jogging or squash as being adequate for the very different purpose we are considering. Of course, a degree of aerobic fitness, achieved by means such as these (or by swimming or cycling or cross-country skiing) is useful to everybody, both for general cardiovascular health and to assist in coping with a second phase of more specific exercises; however, the aerobic phase alone will not suffice. Alongside it, a programme of flexibility and stretching exercises would be ideal. Then, after perhaps six weeks of the aerobic + flexibility routines, relevant strength development should begin. Three visits a week, for six or eight weeks, to a strength-training room or circuit (provided each has upper-body emphasis) would make a great difference, to both efficiency as a crew member and resistance to injury. If rope-pulling is among one's frequent tasks, a weight stack pulled on by a wire, with leg, back and arm involvement, is an excellent preparation. But if winch-handling is one's main duty, nothing but a simulation of the real thing will provide good, specific training.

Boardsailing (ii)

Nature of the Sport

Boardsailing is as far from the sailing of large yachts as the human imagination has yet found it possible to go, while still achieving propulsion across water by the action of air on a sail. Because of their exceptionally high ratio of power to weight (2), sailboards in strong winds can go 2—3 times faster than the largest yacht. These ultra-fast boards ('sinker' boards) are too small even to float if the sailor stands on them in still air; they are kept above the surface, when moving in strong winds, by the hydrodynamic lift of their own bow-waves. Sailing them in such winds involves perpetual dynamic activity (as well as an enviable sense of balance), in contrast to the long sedentary periods, punctuated by occasional bursts of intense action, which are the lot of the yacht crew. Finally, in the opposite conditions, racing boardsailors – having achieved since the 1992 Olympics a special modification of the International Sailing Federation (ISF) racing rules which many dinghy sailors envy – are allowed to fan themselves along, by 'pumping' the sail against a wind that is too light to drive them fast of its own. These racing sailboards are not sinkers!

Heart Rates and Oxygen Uptakes

Fig. 2 shows the heart rate (HR) record obtained from an Olympic boardsailor during a light-wind race. The sailor was a male, aged in his 20's. Mean HR is 182, and blood lactate at the end of the race measured over 12 mmol·l^{-1}. As we shall see in part (iv), high HR alone is not sufficient to give us unambiguous information as to the metabolic demand of an activity. In this instance, however, we have also a strikingly high blood lactate measurement. Taken together, the two values unambiguously indicate dynamic activity involving large muscle groups, of an intensity well above the purely aerobic range.

De Vito et al. (10) have given direct evidence of the respiratory demands in stronger winds, when the sailors' movement would actually be less than in the light-wind pumping conditions of Fig. 2. Recording

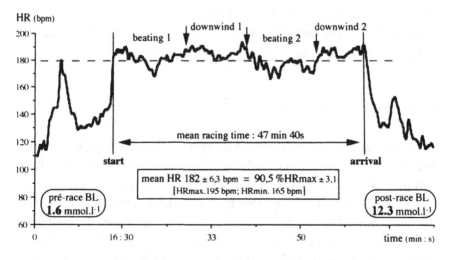

Fig 2 Heart rate record and blood lactate (BL) from an elite boardsailor during French championships. From Gueval et al., J. Sports Sci. 17, 135-141, 1999. With permission.

with the Cosmed K2 telemetric device, these authors found that during-race oxygen consumptions (VO_2) in seven Olympic-level male board-sailors averaged nearly 64 ml·min^{-1}·kg^{-1}. When the same subjects were tested on a cycle ergometer, this value approximately coincided with the breakpoint in their oxygen consumption/workrate plots which has been termed the 'ventilatory threshold' (VT) and normally approximates fairly closely to the lactate threshold (LT). 64 ml·min^{-1}·kg^{-1} is a substantial figure for these thresholds, indicating a high degree of overall aerobic fitness. Nevertheless, is important not to assume an exact match between cycling, which is a lower-body action, and a predominantly upper body activity such as modern boardsailing. Only people who hardly train their legs at all, such as canoeists, reach VT and LT at as high a workrate in an upper body exercise as in a lower body one (27). Appropriately, the blood lactate values recorded on the water by De Vito et al. averaged around 6 mmol·l^{-1}, indicating that the elite sailors studied were working *not at, but well above* LT. Track athletes, in events of similar duration, would have lactates of this order. Allowing for the upper body/lower body comparison, we must not quite equate the two levels of physical demand, but the question asked by the authors, 'Is the Olympic boardsailor an endurance athlete?', should clearly be answered in the affirmative. By the end of a day in which there have been two or even three races, as is normal in international sailing events (but which the 10 km runner would never undertake), the boardsailors' degree of fatigue must be at least as great. Very recent results, using the Cosmed K4 and so including VCO_2 as well as VO_2 data (described by Marchetti in the present volume) underline this conclusion.

Muscular Involvement

In the previous paragraph I took it for granted that modern boardsailing is a predominantly upper body activity. Evidence for this has been given by Buchanan et al. (6). They used a laboratory simulator, consisting of a sailboard hull supported by a waterbed, with the lower part of the mast mounted on the hull by a universal joint and the wishbone boom at its normal height. Weights, simulating different wind forces, acted through the partial damping of a hydraulic buffer. Each of six sailors was required to simulate his/her own actions seen on a video screen, using a film taken previously on water to show both beating and reaching legs of a course sailed in pumping conditions. Surface electromyograms (EMGs) were recorded from up to 13 muscles, and compared with independently studied maximal voluntary contractions (MVCs) of each muscle in turn. Most muscles were even more active during simulated reaching then simulated beating. More importantly, arm and shoulder muscles were typically 2—3 times more active, expressed in terms of % MVC, than leg muscles. Extensor carpi radialis reached a mean in the six subjects of 94% maximal activation during reaching, and biceps brachii averaged over 80% on both points of 'sailing', while four leg muscles (including gastrocnemius and rectus femoris) averaged around 25% of their respective MVCs. The upper body figures were substantially higher than in pre-1992 simulations, for in those not-very-long-ago days boardsailing was an essentially isometric, not dynamic, activity, and was most muscularly demanding in the strongest winds.

The EMG data of Buchanan et al make an interesting comparison with a finding by Bornhauser & Rieckert (5), prior to the 1992 rule change, that forearm muscles swelled painfully during a 5-min static 'hang' from a wishbone, reproducing a problem from which the elite sailors concerned frequently suffered on the water. (It is not clear whether the sailors studied made use of the harness, legalised after the 1984 Olympics, to reduce the isometric load, but the impression from the paper is that they did not.) Almost certainly the mechanism of swelling was osmotic, resulting from accumulation of metabolites within the muscle fibres. It was worst in those subjects with the strongest grip and the greatest forearm circumference; and it was less for every subject in the middle of the sailing season than in winter, when little specific training was apparently then undertaken. Presumably sailing fitness in this respect represented the ability to maintain the same force with less metabolism or more blood flow.

Training for Boardsailing

I meet fewer boardsailors who complain of forearm pain nowadays. Probably two factors have changed as the rules adapted:
a) Sailors have increasingly learned to let the harness take a large percentage of the static body weight off their arms

b) Circulation through dynamically active muscles is much greater than through muscles in constant, more or less static contraction, such as studied by Bornhauser & Rieckert before the 1992 Games.

The first of these proposals is my speculation; the second is undoubtedly true. Nevertheless, Bornhauser & Rieckert arrived at a prescription for dry-land training which would still be on the right lines, for it emphasised multiple-repetition upper body isotonic training with fairly light weights. We can add that circuits and general gymnasium work are also appropriate, with the mean level high in the aerobic intensity range — elevating blood lactate considerably but not exceeding VO_2max. Clearly the percentage time spent on leg work should be a fraction — say 1/3 or 1/4 — of that devoted to the arms, shoulders and back.

Trapezing (iii)

The Two Dinghy Postures

A sailing dinghy floats when stationary, and its mast stands up of its own, not because the sailor holds it up. In both these respects, it differs fundamentally from a sailboard. However, it has no weight beneath the hull. What looks like a keel, its centre or dagger-board, prevents 'leeway' (sideways slippage) but exerts no significant righting moment — indeed in many modern dinghies it is less dense than water, so that when the hull heels the board actually tends to tilt it slightly further. This is the fundamental difference between a dinghy and a yacht.

The consequence is that the crew (one, two, or in a few classes three people) must extend their body weights out over the water to hold the dinghy upright against the wind. In older dinghies this was always done by leaning out, with the feet hooked under 'foot-' or 'toe-straps' near the centre line of the hull — the position known as 'sitting out' or, more recently, for some obscure reason, 'hiking'. Increasingly, however, since the late 1940s, at least the crew and often both/all sailors aboard racing dinghies have been permitted to 'trapeze'. A wire rope, from high on the mast, is clipped to a harness a little above waist level, and the sailor's whole body is suspended outboard, effectively 'standing' horizontally against the top edge of the hull, the 'gunwale'.

Systemic Demands of Trapezing

Trapezing not only exerts greater righting moment than hiking, but it does so with much less physical stress on the crew – provided (s)he is agile enough to move in and out, and fore and aft, as quickly and smoothly as the boat requires. Just how light the physical demands are appears to have been investigated only twice. The one published paper is by Marchetti et al., and dates from 1980 (24). I shall therefore quote also from a student project conducted in my laboratory by Jack, in 1993 (19). Marchetti et al. used just three sailors, but each both trapezed and hiked, and each was studied both in the laboratory and on the water. Jack used 15 subjects, but not all of them for all aspects studied. He simulated static and dynamic trapezing (dynamic, in his experiments = coming in to full knees-bend position and out again, with periodicities in different experiments of 8 and 9 sec). To these he added, in further measurements, the effect of pulling hard on a rope, roughly parallel to the body axis. Both Italian and British subjects were highly experienced, Jack's being mainly members of the Scottish 420 and 470 (trapeze-boat) dinghy squads. Both experimenters examined EMGs, HRs, blood pressures and VO_2 values; Marchetti also included blood lactate.

The two studies agree in concluding that the metabolic and cardio-respiratory demands of steady trapezing are minimal. HR rose just significantly above resting values, typically by about 8 beats per minute(b.p.m) in Marchetti's subjects, 8–18 b.p.m in Jack's. Jack, but not Marchetti, found mean arterial blood pressures significantly elevated: by 30% in static, fully extended trapezing, but no further when a simulation sheet was also being pulled. The diastolic rise was greater than systolic. Both studies found VO_2 values in static trapezing only about 50% greater than at rest, but the values were 250–300% greater ($10 \ ml \cdot min^{-1} \cdot kg^{-1}$) in the dynamic simulations. Marchetti could not detect a significant elevation of blood lactate. Physiologists will recognise this account as typical of low intensity, essentially isometric effort, with a modest dynamic component added in some of Jack's protocols.

Local Muscular Activity

The only divergence between the two studies being discussed (19,24) concerned the identification of which muscles were predominantly responsible for the isometric tone. Considering first the lower body and trunk, Marchetti et al found gastrocnemius (GN) the most active muscle, with rectus abdominis (RA) second but substantially less. Jack found GN less active than thigh muscles he studied (vastus lateralis, rectus femoris) in static trapezing, and none of them displayed more than about 5% MVC, yet RA's activity was about 15% MVC in this position. All values were higher, but in essentially the same sequence, at the fully-extended positions reached during each cycle of dynamic trapezing, RA activation then being more than 25% MVC. Only when the knees were fully flexed did thigh activation exceed that of RA. Probably the differences in straight-body readings between Marchetti and Jack indicate that the Italian subjects trapezed more 'on their toes' than the Scots; the possible influence of different harnesses should not be discounted, but in this instance it was almost certainly secondary.

Turning finally to the upper body, Jack concentrated on the maintenance of sheet tension, which he found required almost 25% MVC activation of biceps brachii, whereas none of the other arm muscles he studied — pectoralis major, deltoid and flexor digitorum longus — significantly exceeded 10% when the subject was fresh. (Rapid fatigue, with activation increasing by the order of 25% in biceps and 50% in the other muscles over the first minute of sustained tension, was a feature of this data set.) Marchetti et al were not concerned with sheeting, but instead made the important finding that the main neck muscle holding the head up, the sternomastoid ('sternocleidomastoid'), was the most active in the body in the simple, isometric posture. This will strike a cord with all trapezers, who often place a hand behind their heads to ease neck strain, and among whose commonest demands upon physiotherapists are those for neck treatment (20). I have wondered whether it would not be worth a manufacturer's while to develop a harness which offers neck support: a simple but well padded rod, extending cranially to take the weight of the head yet not restrict rotation, might make all the difference.

Training for Trapezing

There is no aspect of sailing for which general, gymnasium training is more appropriate than this. For the legs, squat jumps and depth jumps (plyometrics) will be valuable. Those who have large sails to sheet, like assymetric spinnakers, should pull on the weight stack and climb ropes. For sufferers from neck pain, specific neck-strengthening exercises should be regular, with care being taken that not only the flexors but the extensors also are worked upon, to balance the counteracting muscle forces.

Hiking (iv)

Basic Position

Hiking is hard work! With the gunwale beneath some point on one's hamstrings, and all the rest of one's body more or less extended over the water, the load on anterior body muscles is considerable and, for the unfit sailor, rapidly fatiguing and painful. Nevertheless, no competent sailor extends him/herself fully, except in brief periods of particular pressure when maximum righting moment must be exerted. The preferred position is with the spine flexed so that the upper thoracic as well as the cervical region is near vertical (Fig. 3); this posture is much more sustainable, as well as being more appropriate to the 'dagger grip' on the tiller and allowing the head to look around freely. For two or three generations before the present one, a dinghy racer, in a major championship event at sea, might sail in this posture for up to 10 minutes on a single tack. Races are much shorter now, and sailed on smaller courses, so that one tack is unlikely to be held for more than perhaps four minutes — but that is long enough! However, the requirement for hiking may not be confined to the windward legs of a course. The challenge is particularly severe in a large-rig non-trapeze singlehander, such as Laser or Finn, where hiking is required in strong winds on all points of sailing except a dead run.

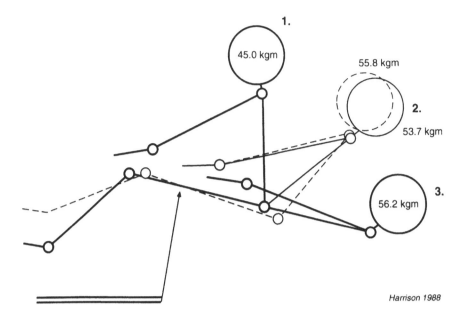

Fig 3 Hiking moments calculated for three main body positions - in this instance, for a young sailor in an Optimist. Position 2 substantially increases the moment, as against position 1, yet position 3 makes only about 5 % further difference at much greater risk of chronic damage to the lower back. If, instead, the toe straps are raised so that the main body weight can be moved outward a little further (dotted position) virtually the same advantage can be achieved much more safely. Courtesy Dr John Harrison.

Biomechanics of Hiking

The preferred posture, described above, which is with spine flexed not hyperextended (kephotic not lordotic) is not only less immediately tiring but substantially less likely to produce long-term damage to the lower back. Documentation of the proneness of sailors to this debilitating problem can be found in many languages (13, 21, 30, 34). For this reason even the fittest sailor should be strongly discouraged from sailing a boat which requires him/her to hyperextend more than very occasionally. As a childrens' coach I have watched in anguish as a light girl, who persisted against my advice on competing against older boys in their preferred class because in skill terms she could clearly match them, suffered ever-worsening lumbar pain until, after three seasons, she had to give up sailing. The dinghy class concerned was the lowly

Topper, but the girl's weight was less than 40 kg while her rivals ranged from 50 to 65 kg — and this was the windy west of Scotland!

The accepted reason (12,16) for the greater long-term safety of the flexed position is that it principally involves the anterior abdominal muscles as the antigravity agonists for the upper body, whereas in the hyper-extended (hollow-backed) position hip flexors, particularly psoas major, are predominantly active. The origin of psoas, on the lower spinal vertebrae, is less robust than that of RA. Furthermore, in bipeds such as ourselves, psoas leads awkwardly over the anterior edge of the pelvis, requiring high tension to achieve the necessary antigravity moment — and the consequence of *this* is that it adds greatly to the compressive force on the lumbar and sacral vertebrae. In further contrast, tension in RA raises intra-abdominal pressure, adding to the surety that the spine will curve kephotically, as it has evolved to do comfortably, and not at any point the other way.

The evidence for these views stems principally from studies of sit-up exercises (12,16), rather than of hiking itself, but there is no reason to distrust it on that account. Furthermore, it is by appropriate use of sit-ups that one can best train the abdominals to dominate the hip flexors, and ensure that one is not inappropriately stressing the lumber vertebrae at the same time. Knees should be bent, feet unrestrained, and head raised before shoulders before thorax — the 'trunk curl' rather than the old-style sit-up, which almost inevitably starts with a hollow back.

Much of the understanding of the abdominal floor exercises, just summarised, comes from EMG studies, and this technique has been among those applied also to hiking itself. Vogiatzis and colleagues (32) have concluded on this basis that the hiking posture on a laboratory simulator, with heavy sheeting, involves quadriceps in contractions between 30 and 40% of MVC, biceps 20-30%, but abdominals only 10-15%. Probably the equivalent values at sea would be intermittently but not constantly higher; however we have not so far found it possible to take the EMG apparatus available to us afloat in the strengths of wind that are of interest. It is desirable that the problems are overcome, because Mackie et al (23), using force transducers in the toe-strap mountings of New Zealand Olympic Finn, Laser and Europe sailors, have concluded that the leg extensors apply average forces in the range 85-96% MVC in winds of 16—18 knots (9—10 m.sec^{-1}). Conversion to %MVC was based on off-water simulations, and I have to say that I am uneasy about the values deduced. Surely not even New Zealand supermen could maintain such mean levels for periods of 30—50 minutes, as the published traces indicate? However, Mackie's data at least suggest that our own laboratory measurements should be considered as representing lower bounds for the on-water loadings. Nevertheless, the crux point is that, if classical physiological observations are correct (1, 22), 30% MVC in a large muscle group is itself sufficient to occlude the muscles' blood flow near-completely. A similar conclusion is reached by Marchetti (this volume). In effect, the dinghy hiker's quadriceps are operating under self-imposed 'tourniquet'. The importance of this will emerge under the next subheading.

Systemic Demands of Hiking

As long ago as 1969, Cudmore[7] used a telemetric pulse rate meter to study the cardiovascular demands of Finn sailing. More recent recordings have given higher values, so that mean HRs from 160[18] to 185[8] b.p.m (Fig. 4) have been reported. In purely cardiac terms, therefore, it has been possible to maintain that a 2.5—3 hour race, such as

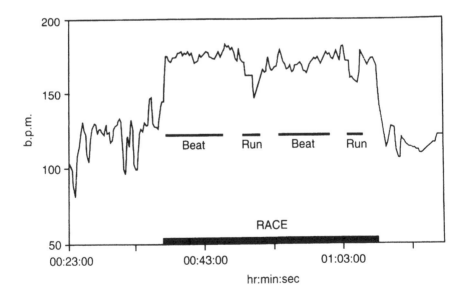

Fig 4 Heart rate record from an elite Laser sailor during a race. Legs marked neither „beat" nor „run" were reaches. Courtesy Mr Peter Cunningham.

might have been sailed in major competitions a generation or two ago, was equivalent to a marathon. The question was, 'Should one train essentially the same way as for a marathon?' (The equivalent model at the turn of the millenium would be a 10-15 km running race.) Those of us who have studied this question scientifically are almost, though not quite, unanimous in answering, 'No'! However, the arguments must be presented with care.

The first experimental indication that extensive aerobic training, of the marathoner's type, would not be appropriate for the dinghy sailor, was by Marchetti et al (24), in the paper previously cited for its parallel study of trapezing: already, in their data, hiking HRs rose far higher than those when the same subject trapezed, *yet VO$_2$ was proportionately much less elevated.* Confirmatory recent results by the Italian group are summarised by Marchetti in this volume. Harrison and colleagues (17), in an investigation which, though confined to the laboratory, was considerably more extensive than the 1980 Marchetti study, compared the same subjects when hiking on an elegantly designed simulator, and when pedalling a cycle ergometer. They found that the oxygen uptake at a given HR was typically about twice as great on the cycle ergometer as on the dinghy one. Other laboratory data pointing to the same conclusion were subsequently obtained by both Vogiatzis (32) and Blackburn (4). The latter used much the same technique to maximise realism as later adopted by Buchanan et al for their boardsailing study – namely, film of a Laser sailor on water, the experimental subjects (all elite Laser helms themselves) being required to mimic the same movements displayed on a screen as they 'sailed' the dinghy ergometer in the lab. Vogiatzis (32, 33), however, also used the Cosmed K2 telemetric system to study VO$_2$/HR relationships in Scottish national squad Laser and Finn sailors during winter race-training at sea. He was able to obtain records in winds of up to 12 m·scc^{-1} (22 knots, or force 6 on the Beaufort scale). HRs in these conditions sometimes exceeded 190 b.p.m., yet no VO$_2$ reading significantly exceeded 30 ml·min^{-1}.kg^{-1}; the overall VO$_2$/HR relationship was only a little steeper than in the lab simulations (Fig. 5). Finally, De Vito et al (9) have also used the Cosmed on water, to make the intesting comparison of Laser dinghy sailors with Mistral boardsailors. Their dinghy results were closely comparable to those of Vogiatzis, whereas boardsailors showed similar HRs but much higher values for VO$_2$ (c.f. section ii).

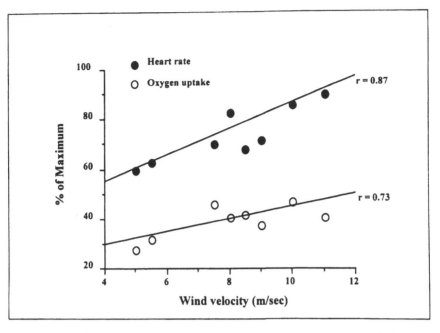

Fig. 5 Effects of wind velocity on heart rates and oxygen uptakes, respectively, in Scottish squad Laser sailors during winter training at sea. Both parameters are expressed as percentages of their maxima, measured on the same individuals using a cycle ergometer. From Vogiatzis, et al. J Sports Med Physical Fitness, 35, 103-107, 1995. With permission.

Quasi-isometric exercise

To the professional physiologist, the explanation for the non-standard VO_2/HR relationship seems obvious. So much of the anterior body wall is under tension for long periods that the HR elevation is that described in classical observations (1, 22) on isometric exercise. The 'purpose' (to speak teleologically) of this high HR is presumably to elevate blood pressure and so force some blood through the vascular beds of self-tourniqueted muscles. However, the relevance of this explanation to truly elite competitors is rejected by some — both coaches and scientists — who are impressed by the highly dynamic nature of such a sailor's performance during a race. In my view, this can make only a marginal difference, for whilst the body is extended above the water, however mobile it may be in this position, the 'tourniquets' are not significantly released. Any improvement of blood flow cannot conceivably approach that obtaining in the relaxed half of every duty cycle during a standard dynamic exercise, such as running or cycling. I have previously described this situation of movement within a period of sustained high load as 'pseudo-isometric', but Dr Stephen Legg employs the better term, 'quasi-isometric'. The point we are both making is that, although the muscles are continually making small adjustments to their length, their *metabolic* situation must be assumed to differ negligibly from that obtaining when they are exactly isometric.

There is, of course, no dispute that the arms and shoulders of all sailors, especially the elite ones, are in vigorous dynamic activity during strong-wind competition. Some of the cardiorespiratory response – probably quite a large part – is elicited by this activity. Even when considering this, however, one should recall the differences between upper and lower body activity (27), already remarked in section (ii). Dynamic upper body work elevates HR disproportionately more than dynamic lower body work, for the same VO_2: the shortfall of oxygen consumption, below what might be naively predicted on the basis of HR, is far less severe than that due to isometric, or even pseudo-isometric exercise, yet the two effects are in the same direction. However, the substantive debate is not about the physiological state of the arms, it is about that of the legs. Is their condition truly dynamic too, in the topmost sailors, or is it even in them pseudo-isometric?

Can we learn anything more from lactate readings? On-water data are a little higher than those obtained in simulations, but they are never very high. Vogiatzis, in the Scottish Squad sailors, rarely got an individual titre above 4 mmol·l⁻¹, and in a linked series (Fig. 6) did not reach this figure. Cunningham, studying the truly elite, has I understand had a few readings around 5 mmol·l⁻¹, e.g. after the race recorded in Fig. 4 the lactate level was 4.8 mmol·l⁻¹ (personal communication). These figures are nowhere near those for boardsailors pumping, but approach those we saw in section (ii) for such sailors in stronger winds. They imply hard effort – but we know hiking is that! The problem is, what sort of hard effort? If, as I believe, most of the anterior body musculature is markedly under-perfused, its metabolism must have a large anaerobic component. Given the vigorous arm work in parallel with this, one should perhaps be surprised the lactates are not higher. (It is not that the lactate is trapped in the muscles, and would be washed out later. For practical reasons, all lactate measurements are made a matter of minutes after the hard hiking has ceased. We are seeing the clearance

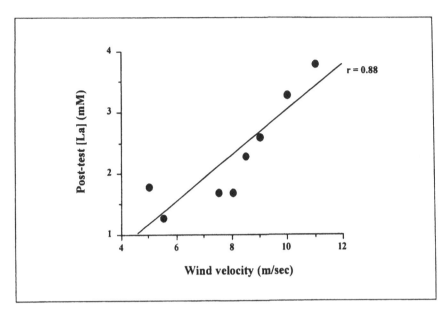

Fig 6 Blood lactate concentrations correlated with wind velocity in the same sailors as for Fig 5. Note that each point is from a different sailor, so the similarity to a typical lactate accumulation curve, as for a single subject in an incremental exercise test, must be viewed with caution. From Vogiatzis, et al. J Sports Med Physical Fitness, 35, 103-107, 1995. With permission.

surge, if there is one to see.) The alternative interpretation, that the elite sailor's whole body is working intensively but dynamically, and so is fully perfused, would be equally compatible with lactate titres in the range observed.

Thus neither HR nor blood lactate is decisive. Only oxygen consumption can resolve the issue of the kind of physiological challenge the hiking sailor meets. We know for Scottish and Italian national-level competitors in training, and Australians of that standard in realistic simulation, that much of the load is quasi-isometric. To maintain that the situation is entirely different in an Olympic final requires the belief that the top few people in the world are not doing the same thing better than those just behind them, or than themselves in experiments and simulations, but doing something entirely different. I know of no other sport where this is true. However, until the complete Olympic Laser fleet agrees to sail the last race wearing Cosmeds, perhaps we shall never really know.

Training for Hiking

The debate just presented is not academic. It has considerable implications for training. The rules of specificity are obvious. If the main demand on the lower body is dynamic, training should be dynamic, but if it is quasi-isometric, training should be quasi-isometric. The former will be based on a substantial volume of aerobic leg activity, grading as the season approaches to intensities above the lactate threshold, plus dynamic strength-endurance work with weights. The second approach will of course not ignore an aerobic base, nor gymnasium exercises to train both arm and hiking muscles (though it is advisable to include in these a proportion of static holds (31)). However, for specific work, the follower of a quasi-isometric programme cannot do better than use the hiking bench, with appropriately-loaded sheeting ropes to train the arms at the same time as the anterior leg and trunk muscles. Yet let it be clear that this bench should not be used purely statically (i.e. strictly isometrically). A past paper from my lab, just cited (31), has caused some confusion as to my view on this: although Burns & I compared purely dynamic with purely static training programmes in our experimental investigation, this was because one needs clear contrasts to do science. The conclusion was that, of the two extremes, static efforts seemed more effective in building *stamina* for the kind of static-plus-dynamic combination which is dinghy sailing. However, these were artificial extremes. Reality must be more complex. In particular, one actually needs speed of response on the water as well as sustained endurance. Thus I do *not* suggest that the way benches were used in the 1960s was correct. People then would pride themselves on hanging still for half an hour, as they read the paper or watched a television programme. This gave them great endurance, but must have slowed their responses to variations of wind, sea and trim. Instead I am sure one should be moving much, if not all, of one's time on the bench. The trunk should be flexing laterally, vertically and torsionally, and one arm or the other pumping its sheet very frequently. Yet it remains the case, as the earliest users of hiking benches like Paul Elvstrøm realised 50 years ago, that *the load should not come off the anterior body wall, so free blood flow through that region will not be restored.*

The leg and trunk training should not, one would now say, be literally isometric. However, if my view of this matter is correct it should, like the sailing itself, be *quasi*-isometric!

References

1. Asmussen, E. Similarities and dissimilarities between static and dynamic exercise. *Circ Res* 48 (Suppl 1), 3—10, 1981.
2. Bethwaite, F. *High performance sailing,* Waterline books, 1993.
3. Bertolucci, LE, DiDario, B. Efficacy of a portable acustimulation device in controlling seasickness. *Aviation Space Envir Med* 66, 1155—1158, 1995.
4. Blackburn, M. Physiological responses during 90 minutes of simulated dinghy sailing. *J Sports Sci* 12, 383—390, 1994.
5. Bornhauser, M, Rieckert, H. Volume changes in forearm-muscles during static work: a study on training effects with windsurfers of the German Olympic team. *Med Sci Res* 21, 881-883, 1993.
6. Buchanan, M, Cunningham, P, Dyson, RJ, Hurrion. PD. Electromyographic activity of beating and reaching during simulated sailboarding. *J Sports Sci* 14, 131—137, 1996.
7. Cudmore, B. Heartbeats. *Yachts & Yachting* Oct 14, 1969.
8. Cunningham, P. Personal communication. 1997.
9. De Vito, G, Di Filippo, L, Felici, F, Gallozi, C, Madaffari, A, Marino, S, Rodio, A. Assessment of energetic cost in Laser and Mistral sailors. *Int J Sports Cardiol* 5, 55—59, 1996.
10. De Vito, G, Di Filippo, L, Rodio, A, Felici, F, Madaffari, A. Is the Olympic boardsailor an endurance athlete? *Int J Sports Med* 18, 281—284, 1997.
11. Felici, F., Ricci, B., de Vito, G., Marini, I., di Fillipo, L., Marchetti, M. Spine loading involvement in offshore sailing. *Med Sci Res* 21, 847—849, 1993.
12. Flint, MM. Abdominal muscle involvement during the performance of various forms of sit-up exercise. *Am J Phys Med* 44, 224—234, 1965.
13. Ghislanzone, R, Cecchini, G, Mennuti, N, Prato, W. Traumatologia dello sport: La colonna vertebrale ed il bacino nei velisti. *Med Sport* 135, 6—10, 1982.
14. Gordon, CR, Ben-Aryeh, H, Spitzer, O, Doweck, I, Gonen, A, Melamed, Y, Shupak, A. Seasickness susceptibility, personality factors and salivation. *Aviation Space Envir Med* 65, 610—614, 1994.
15. Gordon, CR, Spitzer, O, Doweck, I, Shupak, A, Gadoth, N. The vestibulo-ocular reflex and seasickness susceptibility. *J Vestib Res* 6, 229-233, 1996.
16. Hall, SJ, Lee, J, Wood, TM. Evaluation of selected sit-up variations for the individual with low back pain. *J App Sports Sci Res* 4, 42—46, 1990.
17. Harrison, J, Bursztyn, P, Coleman, S, Hale, T. A comparison of heart rate, oxygen uptake relationship for cycle and dinghy ergometry. *J Sports Sci* 6, 160.
18. Harrison, J, Coleman, S. The physiological strain of racing a small, singlehanded dinghy. *J Sports Sci* 5, 79-80, 1987.
19. Jack, ES. A study of the trapezing position in dinghy sailing. *BSc Thesis, University of Glasgow,* 1993.
20. Jones, P. Voyage into uncharted waters. *Physiotherapy in Sport* 11, 3—4

21. le Goff, P. Biomechanique du rachis lombaire at navigation a voile. *Rev Rhumatisme* 55, 411—4, 1988.

22. Lind, AR. Cardiovascular adjustments to isometric contractions: static effort. In: *Handbook of Physiology, sect 2, The Cardiovascular System* III, 26, pp 947-966, 1983.

23. Mackie, H, Sanders, R, Legg, S. The physical demands of Olympic yacht racing.

24. Marchetti, M, Figura, F, Ricci, B. Biomechanics of two fundamental sailing postures. *J Sports Med* 20, 325—332, 1980.

25. Niinimaa, V, Wright, G, Shephard, RJ, Clarke, J. Characteristics of the successful dinghy sailor. *J Sports Med Phys Fitness* 17, 83—96, 1977.

26. Pingree, BJW, Pethybridge, RJ. A comparison of the efficacy of cinnarizine with scopolamine in the treatment of seasickness. *Aviation Space Envir Med* 65, 597—605, 1994.

27. Sawka, MN. Physiology of upper body exercise. In: Pandolph, KB (ed). *Exercise and Sports Science Reviews*, vol 14, pp 175—211, 1985.

28. Shephard, RJ. Biology and medicine of sailing: an update. *Sports Med* 23, 350—356, 1997.

29. Shojaku, H, Ito, M, Watanabe, Y, Mizukoshi, K. Neurotological evaluation of susceptibility to seasickness of inexperienced sailors. *Equilib Res* 53, 482-489, 1994.

30. Simmonet, J. Les problemes rachidiens en voile. *Cinesiologie* 80, 239—242, 1981.

31. Spurway, N.C., Burns, R. Comparison of dynamic and static fitness-training programmes for dinghy sailors - and some questions concerning the physiology of hiking. *Medical Science Research* 21, 865—867, 1993.

32. Vogiatzis, I., Spurway, N.C., Sinclair, J, Wilson, J. The physiological demands of dinghy racing. *Research Report No 40, Scottish Sports Council*, 1995.

33. Vogiatzis, I, Spurway, NC, Wilson, J, Boreham, CJ. Assessment of aerobic and anaerobic demands of dinghy sailing at different wind velocities. *J Sports Med Physical Fitness* 35, 103—107, 1995.

34. von Dierck, S, von Dierck, Th. Belastung und Schadigunsmoglichkeiten des Stutzund Halteapparates bei Seglen. *Deutsche Z Sportmed* 11, 353—361, 1982.

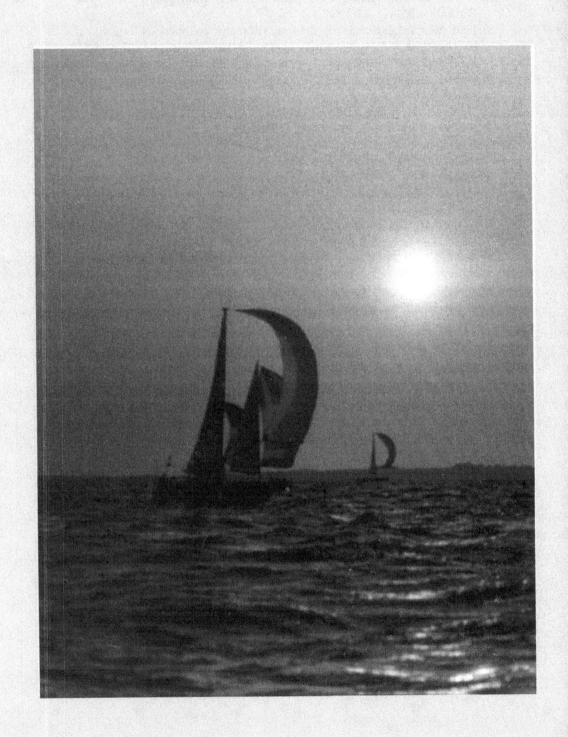

Long-distance offshore sailing race – a nutritional challenge

Leif Hambræus & Stefan Branth

Synopsis

Our observations suggest that a high energy diet plan, including a well planned intake of essential nutrients, e.g. vitamins and trace elements, both during the race and on shore during the brakes for optimal recovery, may be helpful in preserving FFM and restoring energy stores. There is an obvious need for extremely careful planning of the food intake during offshore sailing race in the future for those who intend to win.

Introduction

The impact of nutritional status on physical and psychological performance in athletes is well-known. During the last years much interest has been devoted to the role of an adequate diet and supply of energy and essential nutrients for optimal performance in athletes (7). Experience has shown that there are problems to sustain adequate energy balance which leads to reduced physical capacity and alertness (5, 14). Furthermore, there are indications that there may be an increased demand for certain essential nutrients due to the high energy turnover and especially the stress situations to counteract a potential negative effect of free radicals (2, 17).

Offshore racing
– a recreational exercise or tough athletic performance?

Bernardi and collaborators (1) in their study on offshore boats and using a boat simulator in the laboratory, listed sailing among aerobic *recreational* exercises, based on their findings that the energy output was moderate and blood pressure unchanged, due to the short duration of isometric efforts. However, in their study they were not following the situation under such stress situations as in the Whitbread Around the World Race, neither were the offshore boats of 1990 as extreme as the boats participating in offshore races of today. Their results may thus not be relevant for those participating in the Whitbread Around the World Race, which is considered to be the hardest offshore sailing race in the world, including sailing legs lasting up to 30 days under tough weather conditions, which means a tremendous physiological and psychological stress for the participants.

The physiological and mental stress during offshore sailing depends on many factors, including weather conditions (heavy sea, hard wind), type of craft, navigational problems, tactic decisions and co-operation difficulties within the crew. In addition the watch system with usually 4-h watches and 3-h sleep makes it impossible to get a full nights sleep and causes circadian variations in physical and mental performance.

The modern offshore racing yacht is quite extreme and more similar to a large dinghy than a conventional displacement yacht. This necessitates continuous active muscular work to counterbalance the movements of the boat. Work on deck can sometimes be quite difficult and even dangerous and trimming the sails requires very vigorous sustained contractions of arm muscles. The modern offshore racing yacht thus needs a physically well-trained crew if optimal results should be obtained. An untrained crew member and poor nutrition will definitely impair results and offshore races can no longer be characterised as recreational exercise.

Long-distance offshore sailing race – a nutritional challenge

Offshore racing especially under long periods (several weeks) under tough environmental conditions also represents a nutritional challenge. In addition to a limited availability of fresh food during the race, weight restrictions as well as little storage space, call for light weight products making freeze-dried products a must. The limited water supply, also as a result of weight restrictions, necessitates production of desalinated, low-mineral containing water. Although the biology and medicine of sailing has been discussed (18), there are limited data available regarding the energy needs as well as extra needs for micronutrients, e.g. vitamins and trace elements during offshore racing. The possibilities to study nutritional problems during offshore sailing are, however, unique, as there is a complete control of the food items available and consumed while the crew members are on board.

The risk of development of specific nutritional deficiencies, i.e. vitamin deficiencies like scurvy in the old days when Windjammers were sailing from Australia to Europe, may no longer be a major nutritional problem. Nevertheless Fogelholm and Lahtinen (9) found that the intake of vitamin B_6, magnesium and zinc was marginal in the crew they studied during a transatlantic race. Our findings of reduced magnesium levels in blood and changes in magnesium balance (see below) also indicate that there might be problems of micronutrient imbalances in crew members participating in offshore races.

How to evaluate energy requirements

As stated by FAO/WHO/UNU (8) energy requirements should as far as possible be determined from estimates of energy expenditure. To determine requirements from observed intakes is less accurate as actual intakes are not necessarily those that maintain a desirable body weight and optimal levels of physical activity. Furthermore it is a well-established fact that estimates of dietary intakes by most dietary recall and record methods lead to a 20-30% underestimation of the actual intake (16).

For obvious reasons it is not possible to perform any detailed registration of physical activity throughout an offshore race and it is also impossible to perform heart frequency registrations throughout 25-30 days without interfering with the racing conditions. Any technical equipment would also increase the weight load on board which is not accepted by the racing team. Indirect information about the physical load based on data from the logbook and reports about weather conditions and changes of sails are of limited value. Thus there is limited if any chance to estimate the energy turnover based on conventional methods for estimating energy expenditure. The only other way to estimate total energy turnover is to evaluate the sum of *exogenous* and *endogenous* energy sources. This necessitates not only a careful registration of food consumed, which can be performed at least for the whole crew using food inventories as described below, but also analysis of changes in body composition throughout the race.

Estimations of exogenous energy during offshore racing

One of the advantages with studies on crew members during long-distance offshore sailing is the fact that it offers a unique chance to calculate the food intake with good precision using food inventories. Every food item can thus be registered before and at the end of the competition, i.e. before the boat leaves the harbour and after it has arrived in the new harbour. Leftovers, if any, can be calculated as well as the food items that for one reason or another has been thrown overboard. However, as racing conditions prevent recording individual dietary intakes of the crew members, only the total food intake can be calculated from food inventory records obtained. The total amount of food items consumed can then be used to calculate mean energy and nutrient intake using food tables.

Endogenous energy release indicated by changes in body composition

In order to evaluate the endogenous energy release, changes in the body composition throughout the race has to be studied. This can only be performed by means of anthropometric measurements, i.e. body weight, subcutaneous fat, in combination with various forms of methods in order to estimate body composition.

Doubly labelled water technique offers new possibilities to estimate energy turnover under field conditions

A new approach to estimate energy turnover under field conditions was offered with the introduction of the doubly labelled water technique

(15, 19). This method is extremely well adapted to the conditions during at least shorter offshore sailing legs as the needed time between analysis, although related to the total energy turnover, in this case is about 2 weeks. There is also extremely little interference with the working conditions of the crew, as the only thing needed is to consume the doubly labelled water portion as close to the start of the leg as possible and to collect urinary specimens on at least two occasions after arrival. The only precision that is needed in the sampling procedure, which involves the crew members, is to know that all water is consumed and that the exact time between intake and voiding the urine is recorded.

Performed studies

Fogelholm and Lahtinen (9) studied the dietary intake and nutritional status in a sailing crew during a transatlantic race and reported the mean energy intake to be 13.3 MJ. We have studied the nutritional situation during the two latest Whitbread Around the World Races, 1993/94 and 1997/98, respectively. The first comprehensive study on energy balance and nutritional problems during these offshore sailing race conditions was made by Branth and collaborators during the 1993/94 race and showed a very high energy turnover, 18-20 MJ per day and signs of extensive stress conditions (3). The study was performed on 11 male crew members of the Intrum Justitia team during the first 3 legs of the race (Southampton – Punta del Este, 25 days; Punta del Este - Freemantle, 26 days; Freemantle – Auckland, 13 days).

In the 1993/94 study as well as the 1997/98 study, we were recording the body weight, after overnight fasting and voiding morning urine, before the start as well as at the finish of each leg. Skin caliper measurements were performed as well as bioimpedance measurements and body fat content estimated using the multicompartment model as described by Forslund et al (11).

The study comprised studies on the body composition changes as well as estimations of their food consumption. The food intake registered by means of the inventories was found to be insufficient with respect to energy in most crew members. Thus the mean weight loss was estimated to be around 3 kg during the first leg and somewhat less during the second and third legs. The weight gain during the stopovers,

Table 1. Energy turnover in 6 male crew members during the third leg at the 93/94 Whitbread Around the World Race (the values refer to MJ per 24 hour)

Subject	Energy turnover* (ET)	Endogenous energy** (EE)	Exogenous energy from food inventory***	adjusted (ET - EE)
1	21.7	3.1	16.9	18.6
2	21.7	1.9	16.9	19.8
3	20.1	5	16.9	15.1
4	20.5	2.4	16.9	18.1
5	18.6	2.5	16.9	16.1
6	18.1	3.2	16.9	14.9
Mean	20.1	2.3	16.9	17.1
Total			101.4	102.6

*	estimated by means of doubly labelled water technique
**	estimated from changes in body composition
***	estimated from total food consumption based on food inventories divided by number of crew members

however, seemed to be about the same as the weight losses during the legs.

During the third leg, the energy turnover was also studied in 6 of the crew members using the doubly labelled water technique in order to confirm the calculated energy turnover based on food inventories and changes on body composition (table 1). As shown in this table it was possible to calculate the individual dietary energy intake when total energy turnover was corrected for changes in body composition. Thus it is possible to estimate total energy turnover from the estimation of food intake based on food inventories, compensated by changes in body composition.

A second study was performed during the 1997/98 race on the crew members of the two EF boats, EF Language with a male crew, and EF Education, with a female crew, respectively.

That there is a considerable amount of tissue breakdown as result of negative energy balance was illustrated by the weight losses observed through both Whitbread Around the World Races. During the 1993/94 race it was shocking to see the weight losses of the crew members of the Intrum Justitia team during the first leg (table 2). This however helped to convince those involved of the essentials to better cover

Table 2. Studies on weight changes and energy turnover during the first leg at the 93/94 and 97/98 Whitbread Around the World Races.

	1993/94	1997/98	
No of subjects	11	8 (females)	12 (males)
Mean age (yrs)	33.7	33.9	35.8
Mean body weight (kg)	82.7	84.3	82.6
Mean body fat (%)	20.8	19.6	17.5
Mean BMR (MJ)	7.76	8.23	7.88
Mean weight loss (kg)	3.2	5.6	5.6
Mean energy intake (MJ)	15.0	12.2	12.2
Mean endogenous energy (MJ)	4.5	4.6	4.59
Reference values (FAO/WHO/UNU 1985)			
moderate work (BMR-factor 1.78) (MJ)	13.8	14.6	13.9
heavy work (BMR-factor 2.10) (MJ)	16.3	17.3	16.4

energy and nutrient needs. Nevertheless there were considerable losses in body weight among most crew members and teams during the same first leg at the 97/98 race (table 2). The lack of meal and insufficient energy intake may very well also have determined the outcome of the first leg for some of the boats during the 97/98 race, as discussed by one of the commentators in the Internet discussion (Stephen Pizzo).

The results confirmed our earlier observations that the energy turnover was higher than those observed by Fogelholm and Lahtinen, being around 18-20 MJ. The discrepancy in the estimated energy turnover during offshore racing reported by Fogelholm and Lahtinen in 1991 (13.3 MJ) and that of us during the 1993/94 race (18-20 MJ) may be due to the fact that Fogelholm and Lahtinen only calculated the exogenous energy source. But it may also illustrate that the present offshore races are much tougher than earlier years. This energy turnover level corresponds to that registered in top athletes during training camps, which makes the nutritional demands considerable.

During the 1997/98 race we were also able to study the changes in body composition during the legs as well as stopovers. Of special interest was then to note that there were clear changes in the breakdown and building of fat and muscle tissues during the various legs and recreational stopovers, which might indicate metabolic disturbances as result of the stress condition and energy deficit and call for detailed analysis.

Large magnesium losses

Intracellular magnesium is critical for the production of energy and is intimately associated with adenosine triphosphate concentration and energy utilization (12). In this perspective it is of interest that we observed a disturbed magnesium balance in the crew members as indicated by decreased magnesium levels in blood, e.g. granulocytes, and increased magnesium levels in hair specimens obtained (Fig. 1). Although magnesium is mainly excreted through the urine, increased magnesium levels in hair indicate a constant and large magnesium loss throughout the race, probably as a result of losses from the intra-cellular to the extracellular space, i.e. serum. Energy restriction has only been shown to slightly decrease serum magnesium levels in athletes before (10). Stress caused by physical exercise has, however, been reported earlier to induce hypomagnesiaemia (6) but not as dramatic as shown in our crew members. Interestingly, Fogelholm and Lahtinen (9) reported a low intake of magnesium in their crew members based

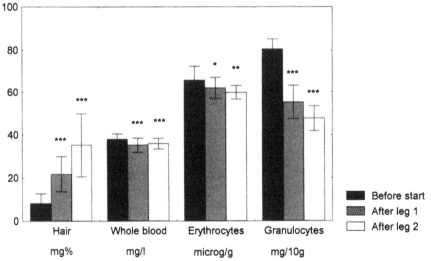

Fig. 1 Magnesium levels in the blood before (Southhampton), and after the first leg (Punta del Este) and second leg (Freemantle). Specimens analysed for hair and whole blood by gaschromotographic methods, and erythrocytes and granulocytes by the PIXE method as described elsewhere (Branth et al, 1998). The changes in relation to values obtained before the start (Southhampton) are significant (* p< 0.05; ** p< 0.01, *** p< 0.001) for all specimens after leg 1 and 2, respectively.
(Please observe that the values are given in various denominations in order to fit into the figure)

on the inventory studies, which might further stress the magnesium balance. The disturbed magnesium balance in our study, however, occurred in spite of the fact that the sailors took daily supplements including 400 mg magnesium. Substantial magnesium losses are otherwise only seen in clinical situations characterised by stress and serious injuries where circulating catecholamines are increased (20). Increased lipolysis when fatty acids are mobilised (13) could also explain decreased magnesium levels in blood occurring during long endurance events at energy deficit, as in our study. The fact that the energy deficit was considerable could thus indirectly be an important contributor for the substantial magnesium losses on a cellular level. It should also be noted that animal experiments have indicated that magnesium deficiency reduces physical performance and in particular the efficiency in energy metabolism (13). Loss of intracellular magnesium can also lead to muscle weakness and neuromuscular dysfunction (4) which agrees with the symptoms experienced by the crew members in the latter part of each leg.

The crew developed signs of deficiencies on several minerals in addition to that described for magnesium, e.g. also losses of zinc were noted. This occurred despite the fact that the crew members were offered a supplementation program including these minerals. A positive effect of magnesium supplementation among exercise persons having low dietary intakes has been reported earlier resulting in increased muscle strength. This might be even more effective in energy deficient situations, although magnesium has been proposed to play an essential role for the protein synthesis leading to preservation of FFM. The potential impact of zinc deficiency on protein synthesis may also have contributed to the muscle losses and has to be taken in consideration.

Conclusion

Our results reveal that there is a high energy turnover during offshore racing which calls for active nutrition counselling during the planning of the meal composition and meal order. Our studies furthermore seem to indicate that food inventories combined with anthropometric measurements to estimate changes in body composition can give valid information about total energy expenditure and energy balance under these conditions. The stress situation both mentally and physically in combination with a metabolic stress secondary to the negative energy balance, may explain the observed changes in magnesium balance which may secondarily lead to disturbances in energy metabolism, muscle weakness and neuromuscular dysfunction. Our results thus illustrate (i) that offshore sailing race is far more demanding than earlier assumed but also (ii) that nutritional studies during such extreme situations is of great scientific interest and may help us to better understand the metabolic stress in other clinical situations. It is obvious that the continuous increase in racing performance calls for much more interest and engagement in the nutritional situation of the crew members as well as for optimal physical training during the stop overs in order to reload and restore the tissue breakdown during the legs.

The situation with a negative energy balance, muscle losses and problems with the micronutrient balance must have influenced the capacity of performance remarkable. Crew members who want to reach optimal performance have to plan the food intake extremely carefully and in advance. Probably more than other groups of athletes due to large practical feeding problems and long-term perspectives as the strenuous performance continues for several weeks. Thus the food composition with respect to energy and nutrient density and balance is of utmost importance. Individual taste preferences and variations of the menu have also to be taken into consideration. Food are often not consumed in proper amounts because of the taste, even though the sailors are hungry. The crew members individual needs, e.g. energy turnover, also have to be identified well in advance before the start in order to make it possible to indivual advice. A team taking their energy and nutritional needs seriously under consideration and planning the diet carefully will have many advantages against its competitors. Optimal nutrition could be the key for victory.

References

1. Bernardi, M, Felici, F, Marchetti, P,: Cardiovascular load in off-shore sailing competition. *J Sports Med phys Fitness* 30; 127-131, 1990.
2. Bello, AZ: Vitamins and exercise – an update. *Med Sci Sports Exerc* 19; 191-196, 1987.

3. Branth, S, Hambraeus, L, Westerterp, K, Andersson, A, Edsgren, R, Mustelin, M & Nilsson, R: Energy turnover in a sailing crew during offshore racing around the world. *Med Sci Sports Exerc* 28:1272-1276, 1996.
4. Brautbar, N & Carpenter C: Skeletal myopathy and magnesium depletion: cellular mechanism. *Magnesium* 3; 57-62, 1984.
5. Brownell, KD, Steen, SN & Wilmore, JH (eds): Eating, body weight and performance in athletes: Disorders of modern society. Philadelphia: Lea & Febiger, 1992.
6. Dolev, E, Burstein, R, Wishnitzer,R, Lubin, F, Chetriet,A, Shefi, M & Deutser, PA: Longitudinal study of Israeli Military recruits. *Magn Trace elem* 10; 420-426, 1991.
7. Economos, CP, Bortz, S & Nelson, ME: Nutritional practices of elite athletes. *Sports Med* 16; 381-399, 1993.
8. FAO/WHO/UNU Expert Consultation: Energy and protein requirements. WHO Techn Rep Ser 724, WHO, Geneva, 1985.
9. Fogelholm, GM & Lahtinen, PK: Nutritional evaluation of a sailing crew during a transatlantic race. *Scand J Med Sci Sports* 1; 99-103, 1991.
10. Fogelholm, GM, Koskinen, R, Laakso, J, Rankinen, T & Ruokonen, I: Gradual and rapid weight loss: effects on nutrition and performance in male athletes. *Med Sci Sports Exerc* 25; 371-377, 1993.
11. Forslund, AH, Johansson, AG, Sjödin, A, Bryding,G, Hambraeus, L & Ljunghall, S: Evaluation of modified multicompartment models to calculate body composition in healthy males. *Am J Clin Nutr* 63; 856-862, 1996.
12. Li, HY, Dai, LJ, Quamme, GA: Effect of chemical hypoxia on intracellular ATP and cytosolic Mg2+ levels. *J Lab Clin Med* 122; 260-272, 1993.
13. Rayssiguir, Y, Guezennec, CY & Durlach, J: New experimental and clinical data on the relationsship between magnesium and sport. *Magnesium Res* 3; 93-102, 1990.
14. Rogers, PJ & Lloyd, HM: Nutrition and mental performance. *Proc Nutr Soc* 53; 443-456, 1994.
15. Schoeller, DA: Measurement of energy expenditure in free-living humans by using doubly-labelled water. *J Nutr* 118; 1278-1289, 1988.
16. Schoeller, DA: How accurate is self-reported energy intake? *Nutr Rev* 48; 373-379, 1990.
17. Sen, CK: Oxidants and antioxidants in exercise. *J Appl Physiol* 79; 675-686, 1995.
18. Shepherd, RJ: Biology and medicine of sailing. An update. *Sports Med* 23; 350-356, 1997.
19. Westerterp, KR, Saris,WHM, van Es, M, TenHour, F: Use of doubly labelled water technique in humans during heavy sustained exercise. *J Appl Physiol* 61: 2162-2167, 1986.
20. Whyte, KF, Addis GJ, Whitesmith, R & Reid, JL: Adrenergic control of plasma magnesium in man. *Clin Sci* 72; 135-138, 1987.

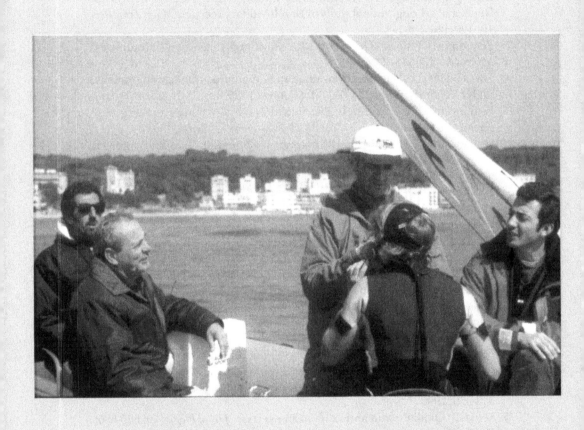

Significance of physiology in tactics choices during sailing

Marco Marchetti

Synopsis

This article regards the possibility of using our knowledge on sailing physiology to optimize Olympic regatta tactics. The muscular effort due to hiking is analyzed as a) energy cost, b) cardiovascular and respiratory stress, and c) local muscular (cellular) fatigue. This latter is considered the central problem and the endurance-force relationship is studied to find the more effective distribution of effort. Nutritional needs are considered also, especially when more than one regatta is scheduled in the day.

The sailing effort

This presentation regards Olympic class only; we will not consider offshore competitions herein. Our concern is the distribution of effort during the race or during the day if more than one regatta is scheduled for the day. The regatta rules have recently been changed and the duration of the competition is now much shorter in comparison with the past. The windward tack especially has been reduced to 15-20 minutes depending on boat and wind speed. In this time the sailor must produce the maximum effort he can maintain until the end of the tack. Furthermore often two or three regattas are scheduled in one day, and the rest time between two competitions can be as short as 10 minutes. What are the possibilities of winning the second regatta if the sailor has strenuously performed during the first? Unfortunately, we have not sufficient information to deal with this question which needs further investigation. Therefore, we had better turn to the following question. What are the local (muscular) and general functional modifications related to regatta fatigue and what are the possibilities of returning to the initial metabolic situation?

Recently Shephard presented an updated review on the Biomechanics and Physiology of small craft sailors (22). The physiology and biochemistry of sailing studies are in their early stages and the following will be more a presentation of problems than a recipe of useful suggestions.

First we need to define effort. Sailing is a very different activity in comparison with other sports. In mild wind and sea athlete fitness is less important than other qualities such as dexterity in rudder and sail trimming, knowledge about meteorology and regatta rules, and tactic competence. The sailor's fitness becomes increasingly relevant when wind speed increases. This special quality is often related to endurance in hiking. To counteract the wind's capsizing effect the sailor projects himself out of the boat. Proper hiking is performed when no trapeze is used for sustaining the upper part of the body. The exercise involves deck instep support plus the boat board for posterior thigh surface

Table 1 Cost of sailing

Olympic class gender	Oxygen intake ml kg^{-1} min^{-1}	Hart Rate. beats min^{-1}	Expiratory Ventilation l min^{-1}
Tornado (males) [*]	11	112	//
Star (forward males)[*]	11	115	//
Star (helmsman males)[*]	10	151	//
Finn (males)[*]	20	106	//
Mistral (males)[**]	43	167	107
Mistral (female)[**]	30	168	65
Laser (males)[**]	22	138	46
Mistral (males)[**]	42	169	108
Laser (males)[***]	20	145	

[*] 11: [**] 6: [***] 8

support. This taxes, by an isometric effort, mainly the abdominal, ileo-psoas and quadriceps muscles (17). Eight or nine different kinds of boat classes participate in the Olympic games, with one, two, or three sailors per boat. Out of a total of 18 sailors (male and female) who compete in different regattas, 11 adopt a variant of the hiking posture. This is the only sport in which the essential component of the performance is a static effort. The sailor's posture is not only static, him having to adapt to waves and wind variation. Thus, on a background of isometric contraction, the sailor must abruptly increase the effort approximating his Maximum Voluntary Contraction (MVC) (7). Furthermore, the sailor must work at hauling aft the sail (jib or spinnaker). Steering also imposes additional work. In a special Olympic class — the Mistral — hauling aft has become particularly heavy exercise since pumping was allowed (4, 6, 8). That is a manoeuvre in which the athlete pulls and pushes the sail in a rhythmic fashion. In this way the sail, acting as a wing, provides additional propulsion to the board.

The energy cost

We can analyze the sailing effort for metabolic energy cost, cardiorespiratory work load and muscular fatigue. The energy cost is a common way of defining performance in Sport Physiology. It is measured assessing the oxygen intake (VO_2), carbon dioxide output (VCO_2) and blood lactate (BL). This has been done in the laboratory using sailing simulators (3, 25, 26) and during actual sailing (6, 8, 11, 27). In both cases the data was compared to the athlete's maximum potential, that is, the maximum aerobic power (VO_2max) and anaerobic threshold (3, 6, 8, 20). The use of K2 portable metabolimeter was found very useful for these measures, especially during actual sailing (6, 8, 11, 27). It teletransmits data on line to a receiving apparatus, which can be kept in a convenient boat. We can obtain VO_2 as well as pulmonary (expiratory) ventilation (EV) and heart rate (HR) data every 15 or 30 seconds. With the more recent K4 metabolimeter VCO_2 is also measured. Finally blood lactate is measured taking a sample of blood from the ear lobe. Data obtained at sea, during regatta simulations, are shown in Table 1. Evidently results obtained by different authors are consistent: A typical figure in dinghy sailing for O_2 intake is about 20 ml per minute and per kg of body mass. Vogiatsis (27) demonstrated that the energy cost

Table 2 Physiological characteristic of sailors

Olympic class gender	Max aerobic power ml kg^{-1} min^{-1}	Heart Rate. beats min^{-1}	V O$_2$ Threshold l min^{-1}
Laser (males) *	62.3	189	//
Mistral (males) **	63.6 $\pm$ 2.3	185 $\pm$ 16	48.5 $\pm$ 3.8
Mistral (females) **	49.2 $\pm$ 4.1	184 $\pm$ 8	30 $\pm$ 4.4
Laser (males) ***	53.4 $\pm$ 3.5	184 $\pm$ 9	38 $\pm$ 5.9
Laser (males)****	52 $\pm$ 6	196 $\pm$ 6	//

* 3; ** 8; *** 6; **** 27

was strictly dependent on the wind velocity. This simply means that the more the capsizing effect of the wind, the more the work requested from the sailor to balance the boat. Comparing the data obtained at sea with the ergometric test it became evident that the energy cost measured at sea corresponded to 1/3 - 1/2 of the maximal aerobic power of the subjects. Physiological characteristics are shown in Table 2. The values measured at sea were well below the anaerobic threshold. Thus the aerobic power request did not result a limiting factor in performing the regatta. However we should consider the possibility that throughout a day (or days) the energy reserve could be depleted to an extent sufficient to compromise the last competition. McLoughlin (18) demonstrated that a reduction in glycogen stores impaired sailing performances.

Nowadays a Laser regatta lasts 50-60 mins. In this time we can estimate a 50-100 g glycogen breakdown. Not a very great amount in comparison with other sports, but we must consider that this loss is mainly at the expense of quadriceps that sustain the greatest torque (7, 17, 21). Furthermore glycogen is the main fuel in an anaerobic – or quasi-anaerobic – condition. The loss of muscular glycogen storage can have a substantial effect if another regatta follows the first with a very brief restoration time of some 15 mins. In this time it is improbable that lactate will be completely removed from the blood and the glycogen muscular storage refilled. When a third regatta is scheduled in the day, the situation can be very dramatic and the athlete can consider the best way to distribute his metabolic reserves throughout the day.

Evidently it depends on strategy considerations and to the possibility to forecast weather conditions. As a general rule, the statement that a competent yachtsman must always do all she/he can in each race maintains all its weight. This aspect assumes particular relevance in the Mistral class. We must remark that it is in light weather that Mistral pumping becomes heavy exercise, because it is in such conditions that pumping is really required. Indeed, in such conditions the boat speed is more than doubled when the pumping effect is added to the wind propulsion. De Vito (6, 8) demonstrated that this activity represents a very heavy energy demanding work. In Mistral athletes they measured 40 ml min^{-1} kg^{-1} VO_2. The laboratory tests demonstrated that these sailors presented the characteristics typical of aerobic athletes (more than 60 ml min^{-1} kg^{-1} VO_2max). De Vito's results revealed that the energy requirement often went above the anaerobic threshold. These data have been recently confirmed on some of the best international athletes by comparing the VO_2 and VCO_2 data obtained with and without pumping (personal data). When Mistral sailing was performed without pumping the oxygen demand was very low. Conversely with pumping it approximated the aerobic maximal power. The VCO_2/VO_2 ratio and the blood lactate confirmed that the anaerobic threshold had been passed. Mistral regattas are very brief, but we can calculate that a 40 minute regatta could result in a 150 gram glycogen loss (8). Quickly absorbed food will be supplied, but it is very doubtful that the glycogen storage can be refilled during the brief interval between two regattas. This problem assumes dramatic relevance when a third regatta has to be sailed in the same day. The above data must be carefully taken into account when assigning the appropriate glycidic and calorie requirements. Furthermore, the data confirm that the rules that limit the number of regattas in a day, and require a 20 min minimum interval between two regattas, are sensible.

Muscular fatigue

With the laboratory simulators the biomechanics of hiking have been extensively studied (3, 7, 17, 21, 25, 26). The greatest torque was measured at the knee, hip and lumbosacral joints. To carry out these measures, a number of very similar boat simulators were designed. We must remember that actual sea conditions cannot really be simulated in the laboratory. On the other hand, meteorological conditions are so unpredictable, that a laboratory environment is preferred if all variables have to be controlled. Furthermore, with the laboratory simulators we can accomplish measurements that are unrealizable in real sailing.

According to recent regatta rules, the windward tack can be performed in less than 20 min. During this time the sailor, in windy conditions, must apply the maximum hiking torque he is able to maintain for the set time. Evidently, local muscular fatigue is the main factor limiting the performance. Recent research has been aimed at studying muscular hiking fatigue, the relationship between hiking torque and endurance, and the effect of hiking on cardiac and pulmonary systems.

Local muscular fatigue was studied with a laboratory simulator when the athlete performed bouts of hiking contractions with a very brief rest interval (26) or a single contraction maintained until exhaustion (3). The inverse relationship between the possibility of maintaining an isometric effort and the intensity of the effort have been quantitatively

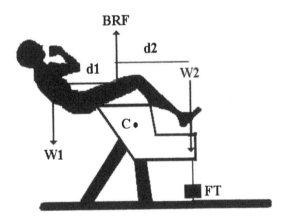

Fig. 1 Schematic representation of the hiking simulator adopted in our experiment (Harken It.). W1 is the force of gravity of the sailor's upper part of the body (Head + trunk + arms = UB). The bench that supports the sailor is a real section of Laser boat, suspended by the pivot C, which simulates the center of water pull on the boat. A force W2 is balancing the torque exerted by the boat and by the sailor. The force transducer FT measures this torque. The sailor is adopting the typical hiking posture to exert the maximum balancing torque. The sailor hooks the feet under straps attached to the bottom of the boat and stretches his upper part of the body (UB) out the board. Respect to simply sitting on the board, he exerts a supplement of torque, equal to the weight of UB times the distance d1. When exerting the maximum torque in this position, generally a fraction of quadriceps MVC is used.

described since the pioneering studies of both Ikay and Rohmert (1). These authors stated that the curve that relates force with endurance (the maximum time the set force can be maintained) is a hyperbolic relationship, similar to the classic force-velocity Hill curve. We requested 8 good Laser athletes to maintain hiking torque (HT) at different percentages of the maximum until complete exhaustion (personal data). The boat simulator used was the one depicted in Fig. 1 (Harken, Italy). In this apparatus the athlete can apply the same isometric HT that he uses to balance the boat during real sailing. This means, as explained in the caption of Fig. 1, that the athlete, when performing the maximum HT (HTmax), is using only a fraction of quadriceps MVC. The athletes were requested to apply 100%, 85% and 60% of HTmax until exhaustion. Plotting the data on a graph, we obtained the distribution shown in Fig. 2. To fit the data we adopted the equation used by Mannion and Dolan (16). These authors used it to fit the force-endurance relationship measured in quadriceps during isometric contractions in sedentary individuals. Correlation tests indicate that our data matched the curve with good statistical significance (P <0.01). These results could be of use. Spurway (23) has stressed the importance of specific isometric training for sailors. The assessment of each athlete's curve can be useful to follow the effectiveness of a training program.

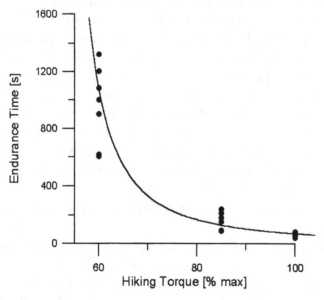

Fig. 2 Endurance torque relationship measured using the experimental setup of fig. 1. Dots refer to individual data.

Acute muscular fatigue is an important topic in exercise physiology, but regarding sailing sports these studies are at their very beginning. We can exclude that a depletion of the local glycidic reserve could be the cause of fatigue, at least in the first minute of hiking exercise. This can be inferred by the previously mentioned studies on energy cost during actual sailing. The measurements we took during hiking simulation confirm this statement. The laboratory simulation demonstrated that energy cost of hiking performed as a simple static exercise (without compensation for waves and wind and without steering or hauling) is very low if compared with other human exercise. Table 3 shows the

Table 3 Energy cost of hiking (personal data)

Hiking at 85% HTmax			Hiking at 60% HTmax		
Energy cost (KJ)	Glycogen equivalent (g)	performance duration (s)	Energy cost (KJ)	Glycogen equivalent (g)	performance duration (s)
47 ± 11	2.8 ± 0.75	189 ± 75	188 ± 78	5.7 ± 2.1	896 ± 313

data we obtained in Laser athletes during hiking at two percentages of maximum torque (HTmax). Evidently the power request is even less than the one measured during actual sailing. Glycogen depletion was also very limited. The glycogen content in well-trained athlete's quadriceps was estimated to be around 14 g kg^{-1} wet muscle weight (12). An athlete 1.8 m tall and 69 kg weight (the mean anthropometric data of our subjects) would have a quadriceps mass for each thigh of 3 kg (13). Even assuming that quadriceps alone contributed to energy supply, and this supply was obtained from glycogen only, 11 out of 84 g total glycogen availability would be a very small intake. Blood lactate was about 4 mmol@l^{-1} as a maximum that indicates a very limited oxygen debt, below the anaerobic threshold. Our data are in accordance with the data previously published in research on hiking simulation (3, 25, 26). In brief, from a metabolic energy point of view, hiking must be considered very light exercise, quite equivalent to level walking at moderate speed.

The most impressive effect of hiking both in laboratory simulation (3, 7, 17, 25, 26) and during actual sailing (6, 8, 11, 17, 27) was the increase in heart rate (HR) and in arterial pressure (AP). Gallozzi[11] noted the great disparity between the increase in HR and the relatively low energy cost of sailing. He assumed that the high HR, observed on a calm day regatta, was entirely due to the emotional stress. While that could be the main cause of cardiac adjustment when very low hiking effort is requested, we must admit that other effects operate when the hiking demand increases. The general effect of static effort has been extensively studied and it is well established (15) that the resistance to blood flow in the muscular vascular bed increases when the force becomes greater than 20% of the MVC. When the muscular contraction is above 50% of MVC the muscle becomes completely ischemic and its metabolism is deeply affected. Many chemicals accumulate in the interstitial fluid and stimulate sensors that send signals to the central nervous system. The first effect is pain that becomes greater and greater with time. At the same time, the stimulation of pontine and medullar cardiovascular control centers elicits a sympathetic volley on the heart that increases the HR. This, in turn, enhances the cardiac output and the paramount effect is the arterial blood pressure greatly increasing. The increase in cardiac output is not compensated for by a corresponding decrease in peripheral resistance, which, conversely remains unchanged. The reflex effect also involves respiratory centers, which make the pulmonary ventilation increase.

All these effects have been deeply studied in human beings and animals and in many experimental conditions. The research previously mentioned indicates that a similar effect is produced in the same way in the sailor during hiking. In the laboratory, albeit using the simulator, the increase in blood pressure was measured with a sphygmomanometer. In our laboratory direct aortic catheterisation confirmed this effect (personal data). Despite having no records of blood pressure during actual sailing, we can be confident that this effect is produced in many instances. Vogiatzis (25, 26) stressed the fact that during Laser sailing pulmonary ventilation increases to an extent that is not justified by the increase in VO_2, VCO_2. The author studied this effect very deeply during bouts of effort with the hiking simulator. He assumed that the hyperventilation was elicited by some chemicals which accumulated in the muscles and there stimulated chemoreflexes. In addition, the increase in efferent neural activity, descending from higher centers to exercising muscles (central command), could diffuse to both cardiac and respiratory centers. Thus the same cause that induced an increase in blood pressure, was active in producing the ventilatory effect (26).

Table 3 shows the data recorded in the same Laser sailors as in table 2. Of particular interest for judging the cardiac work is the double product. This is the product of the mean arterial pressure (MAP) times HR. As illustrated in table 3, we obtained a double product three times greater than at rest. The augmented double product we measured indicates relevant heart work, disproportional to the energy cost of the exercise. A more precise measure of cardiac work could be obtained when the product of MAP times cardiac output is calculated. We did not measure cardiac output during hiking simulation, but an evaluation of this data can be obtained by comparison with other experimental conditions. During isometric effort at 75% MVC, we measured, by cardiac catheterisation, a cardiac output increase to 7-8 l min^{-1}. If a similar increase is assumed during hiking, the cardiac work will correspond to 138 mm Hg times 8 l min^{-1}. This means that cardiac work was 2.5 W whereas rest value was about 1 W. The cardiac work became about 150% greater than rest value. It is noteworthy that this extra cardiac work is mainly due to an increase in pressure. Sport cardiologists are aware of the possible danger inherent in this special cardiac work. This fact must be considered when a medical check up is given to a sailor with the purpose of judging his eligibility for sport. On the other hand, we are confident that this is not such great extra work as to affect the sailor's endurance. Recent research studied the echocardiographic effect of sailing in top level athletes (20). It confirmed that the morphological adaptation to high pressure work consisted of a very moderate hypertrophy of the cardiac wall.

Electromyography

Vogiatzis used the surface electromyography (sEMG) to obtain an insight into the cause of hiking fatigue (25). He described a shift toward the left in the power spectrum frequencies of sEMG. The analysis in the frequency domain is consistently used to detect the first sign of fatigue during isometric effort (9). It is well known that the power spectrum of sEMG becomes progressively modified during the effort, the lower frequencies becoming dominant (19). This is reflected in the progressive decline of the Median Frequency that is considered the best representative of the whole spectrum. This effect was interpreted as a reduction in conduction velocity of action potentials (19). More recently, some authors considered the possibility that this effect was also related to a synchronization of motor unit (MU) activity (14). This could be a special strategy the nervous control center exerts to compensate for the loss of some MUs (probably type IIA MU) which are completely exhausted by the exercise. A possible interpretation is that, to maintain the force despite the reduced number of active MUs, nervous centers reduced all desynchronizing inibitory circuits (e.g., Renshaw neurons). Recently Votgiatsis (26) observed a decline of the Median frequency during a series of hiking bursts and this was confirmed by us during continuous effort endured until exhaustion (personal data).

During hiking Vogiatzis (26) observed an increase in the Root Mean Square of the EMG signal, and that was another evident modification of sEMG correlated with development of fatigue. He attributed this effect to the recruitment of additional MUs to compensate for the force reduction in fatigued MUs. Recently Bernardi (2) observed this sEMG modification during increasing isometric effort, and explained this effect as the combined contribution of the increase of MUs firing rate and recruitment. In our opinion the same interpretation can be assumed in hiking fatigue too. Hypotheses aside, we consider that all the above techniques reveal a definite trend during effort that is an early indicator of developing fatigue. In Fig. 3 an example of sEMG and of integrated EMG we obtained during hiking simulation is shown. Their study could prove useful in following the progress of training in future sailors.

As a determinant of muscular pain induced by fatigue, K^+ is the main candidate (3, 26) among other factors like H^+ and Lactate. Its accumulation in the interstitial fluid of the muscle is due to the outflow from repolarisizing fibers. This could be effective in sending afferent signals to the central nervous system to induce pain. They could induce the cardiovascular and respiratory effect previously described. On the other hand, the K^+ accumulation in the interstitial fluid must be accompanied by a decrease in intracellular K^+ concentration. The resulting reduction in the K^+ gradient across the fiber membrane could produce cell depolarization, a reduced action potential amplitude and in some fibers, complete inactivation (10). Thus K^+ play an important role among the cellular determinants of fatigue. Numerous human studies have observed an increase in plasma K^+ during exercise (10). Conversely, Stieglitz (24) demonstrated that 15 min after a regatta the blood concentration of this ion is deeply diminished. This effect is quan-

LEFT RECTUS FEMORALIS - 80% HT

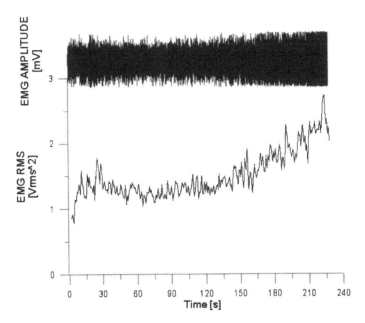

Fig. 3 Upper trace: sEMG recording during hiking maintained until exhaustion; Hiking torque: 80% of maximal hiking torque.
Lower trace: sEMG time domain analysis (Root Mean Square value) of the upper trace.

titatively related to the difficulty of the performance and the fatigue felt by the sailors. The author suggested that the decrease in serum K^+ after a prolonged rest period was due to rapid re-entry of the ion in the skeletal and cardiac muscle cells, previously depleted during the high intensity work. Thus, the post activity serum K^+ could serve as indirect measures of muscular intracellular impairment. Research on the ions imbalance in body fluids during and after a regatta will be of great relevance for developing new regatta strategies.

In conclusion we must admit that the inferences we can offer to improve the sailor's tactic are very elusive. We have just raised the problem and illustrated the relevance. It can be hoped that future research will offer better answeres. Finally, we must remember that the great majority of physiology studies applied to dinghy sailing are limited to two Olympic classes: Laser and Mistral. We definitely need to extend our knowledge to the other classes, with two or three men who could use trapezes instead of hiking and spinnakers instead of jibs.

References

1. Åstrand, P.O., Rodahl, K. *Textbook of work Physiology.* McGraw-Hill Book Company. New York 1970.
2. Bernardi, M., Solomonow, M. Nguyen, R.V. et al. Motor unit recruitment strategy changes with skill acquisition. *Eur J Appl Physiol* 74, 52-59, 1996.
3. Blackburn, M. Physiological responses to 90 min of simulated dinghy sailing. *J Sport Sci* 12, 383-390, 1994.
4. Bornhauser, M., Rieckert, H. Volume changes in forearm-muscles during static work: a study on training effects with windsurfers of the German Olympic team. *Med Sci Res* 21, 881-883, 1993.
5. Cerquiglini, S., Felici, F., Figura, M., et al. Cardiovascular effects of arms wrestling. *Int J Sport Card* 3, 94-102, 1986.
6. De Vito, G., Di Filippo, L., Felici, F., et al. Assessment of energetic cost in Laser and Mistral sailor. *Int J Sport Cardiol* 5, 55-59, 1996.
7. De Vito, G., Di Filippo, L., Felici, F, et al. Hiking mechanics in Laser athletes. *Med Sci Res* 21, 859-860, 1993.
8. De Vito, G., Di Filippo, L., Felici, F, et al. Is the Olympic boardsailor an endurance athlete? *Int J Sport Med* 18, 281-284,1997.
9. Felici, F., Colace, L., Sbriccoli, P. Surface EMG modifications after eccentric exercise. *J Electromyogr Kinesiol* 7, 193-202, 1997.
10. Fitts, R H Cellular mechanism of muscle fatigue. *Physiol Rev* 74, 49-94, 1994
11. Gallozzi, C., Fanton, F., De Angelis, M, et al. The energetic cost of sailing. *Med Sci Res* 21, 851-853, 1993.
12. Hultman, E, Bergstoem, J., Roch-Norlund, A.E. Glycogen storage in human skeletal muscles. In: B Pernow and B Saltin (eds.). *Muscle metabolism during exercise,* pp 273-288, 1970.
13. Jones, M. R., Pearson, J. Anthropometric determination of leg fat and muscle plus bone volume in young male and female adults. *J Physiol* 219, 63P, 1969.
14. Krogh-Lund, C. Myoelectric fatigue and force failure from submaximal static elbow flexion sustained to exhaustion. *Eur J Appl Physiol* 63, 389-401, 1993.
15. Lind, A. R. Cardiovascular adjustments to isometric contractions: static effort. In: *Handbook of Physiology. Section 2. The Cardiovascular System III* pp 947-966, 1983.
16. Mannion, A.F., Dolan, P. Relationship between myoelectric and mechanical manifestations of fatigue in the quadriceps femoris muscle group. *Eur J Appl Physiol* 74, 411-419, 1996.
17. Marchetti, M., Figura, F., Ricci, B. Biomechanics of two fundamental sailing posture. *J Sports Med Phys Fitness* 20, 325-332, 1980.
18. McLoughling, E., Hale, T., Harrison, J.H.H. et al. The effects of dietary manipulation on physiological responses to a 30 minute sailing task. *Med Sci Res* 21, 869-870, 1993.

19. Merletti, R., Knaflitz, M., De Luca, C. J. Myoelectric manifestations of fatigue in voluntary and electrically elicited contractions. *J Appl Physiol* 69, 1810-1820, 1990.

20. Rodio, A., De Luca, R., Sbriccoli, P. et al. Functional and echocardiographic evaluation of Olympic-class sailors. *Int J Sport Cardiol* 5, 105-108, 1996.

21. Schonle, C. Pain and joint stress in sailing. *Med Sci Res* 21, 875-880, 1993.

22. Shephard, R.J. Biology and medicine of sailing. An update *Sport Med* 23, 350-356, 1997.

23. Spurway, N.C., Burns, R. Comparison of dynamic and static fitness-training programmes for dinghy sailors - and some questions concerning the physiology of hiking. *Med Sci Res* 21, 865-867, 1993.

24. Stieglitz, O. Fatigue and serum potassium in high performance sailors. *Med Sci Res* 21, 855-858, 1993.

25. Vogiatzis, I,, Roach, N.K. . Trowbridge.E.A. Cardiovascular, muscular and blood lactate responses during dinghy 'hiking'. *Med Sci Res* 21, 861-863, 1993.

26. Vogiatzis, I., Spurway, N.C., Jennett, S., et al. Changes in ventilation related to changes in electromyograph activity during repetitive bouts of isometric exercise in simulated sailing. *Eur J Appl Physiol* 72, 195-203, 1996.

27. Vogiatzis, I., Spurway, N.C., Wilson, J., et al. Assessment of aerobic and anaerobic demands of dinghy sailing at different wind velocities. *J Sports Med Phys Fitness* 35, 103-107, 1995.